T0046949

The
Fragile
Years

The Fragile Years

Proven Strategies *for the* Care *of* Aging Loved Ones

Amy Cameron O'Rourke

A POST HILL PRESS BOOK
ISBN: 978-1-64293-946-0
ISBN (eBook): 978-1-64293-947-7

The Fragile Years:
Proven Strategies for the Care of Aging Loved Ones
© 2021 by Amy Cameron O'Rourke
All Rights Reserved

Cover art by Cody Corcoran

Although every effort has been made to ensure that the personal and professional advice present within this book is useful and appropriate, the author and publisher do not assume and hereby disclaim any liability to any person, business, or organization choosing to employ the guidance offered in this book.

No part of this book may be reproduced, stored in a retrieval system, or transmitted by any means without the written permission of the author and publisher.

Post Hill Press
New York • Nashville
posthillpress.com

Published in the United States of America
3 4 5 6 7 8 9 10

This book is dedicated to my mom and dad
and my beloved Hobey.

Contents

Contents

Chapter One

A Crisis for the Aging Like No Other

This case began, as so many do, with a frantic call from a loved one.

My husband is in an acute care hospital in Orlando. He is on a ventilator and getting dialysis. They called and said they are discharging him, and the only place that would take him is a nursing home more than five hours away, in Georgia. My lawyer told me to call you. What can I do to stop them from sending him so far away to another state? Can you help me?

As an advocate for aging and fragile clients and their families, I deal with these situations every day. Hospitals do not want to care for long-term patients, especially those on ventilators. It is not cost-effective for them to have a hospital bed tied up for that long with a patient whose condition is unlikely to improve. They are not paid to maintain the care of a patient, only to "cure them."

That is the economics of the situation from the hospital's point of view. I have a different point of view. My job is to fulfill the wishes of my clients and make sure they get the best possible care for the best quality of life in the time they have remaining.

I am in the profession of Aging Life Care Management™, which means I handle similar cases on a daily basis. All too often, hospitals announce that they are discharging fragile patients to places that are far from family because they claim there are no facilities that will take them. And sometimes, that is true.

Hospital discharge directors aren't evil people. They have very difficult jobs governed by numbers, not by emotions. I don't attack them or threaten them in these situations. I offer to work with them to find a better solution. And I know that *they* know this: hospitals and skilled nursing facilities must ensure a safe discharge of their patients. So, the law is on my side.

My first words to the discharge staff member in this case were: "This patient's wife lives in Orlando. She is not moving to Georgia, and her husband is not going to Georgia. Based on what his wife has told me, he may be dying, and if that is the case, he is not going anywhere until our nurse care manager can assess his condition and determine whether it is safe to move him. You might be mad at me now, but you and I are going to become best friends as we work out a nice discharge plan. Rest assured, we will become friends."

Hospital discharge staff members often do get frustrated and angry if anyone interferes with their discharge plans for patients. They consider such people to be a barrier. The discharge staff members are under a lot of pressure to clear out unprofitable patients who are at risk of dying.

My carefully chosen words were the equivalent of saying "checkmate" in a game of chess. Once a family member or advocate questions the safety of moving a patient, the hospital must give them time to evaluate the patient's condition and find a safe place for that person to go.

Now, this case was more complicated than most due to the timing. This occurred in March of 2020. We were experiencing the first wave of the Covid-19 pandemic, which made an already difficult situation about one hundred times more difficult.

As everyone knows by now, the coronavirus hit nursing homes and other long-term care facilities for the aging harder than anywhere else.

"Residents of long-term care facilities constitute less than 1 percent of the U.S. population, yet 43 percent of all COVID-19 deaths through June occurred in those places. The number has changed little since," according to an AARP report, which said there were more than one hundred thousand deaths caused by the coronavirus among residents and staff of US long-term care facilities between March and Thanksgiving of 2020.

In the spring and summer of 2020, I joined my colleagues in Care Management across the nation and worldwide as we had to make a dramatic shift. We went from serving as advocates for older adults to being more like special forces combatants at war. Our enemy was this highly contagious virus that was particularly deadly for our fragile clients.

Nursing homes went into lockdown during the pandemic, and rightfully so—no visitors, including their family and their advocates like me and my team. Many people called me during this period because they were upset that they could not visit their family members in nursing homes.

My stance was always to support the nursing home administrators who were trying to protect all of their residents and staff members from being infected with the virus.

To help our clients and their families, my team took on a new role in addition to our usual responsibilities. We became like the Geek Squad at Best Buy or the Apple store. We trained many people on how to use FaceTime, Zoom, Houseparty, and other apps to communicate remotely with their loved ones and their caregivers inside the facilities during the quarantine. We also dropped off laptops, iPads, and other devices at nursing homes for clients who did not have their own.

There was no preparing for a crisis like the pandemic. We handled it case by case, minute to minute, hour to hour, day to day, as best we could. We juggled many duties, many clients and families, and fought many battles.

Some we lost. Some we won.

My team did manage to keep the Orlando hospital from sending the dying man to Georgia, far from his wife and family. He did not have the coronavirus, but his final days were definitely impacted by it, just as so many others were.

This gentleman was seventy-eight years old, and he'd had a stroke on the golf course. His partners called 911, and doctors resuscitated him in the ER, but the poor guy never regained full consciousness.

After I was called in as the family's advocate, my team had intense conversations with the hospital. I managed to get my company's care manager, Valerie, a registered nurse, inside to evaluate his condition.

After seeing him, Valerie could not understand why they wanted to discharge this patient and have him transported to Georgia. He was basically on life support with a ventilator. She believed that any attempt to move him would result in his immediate death. We also had doubts that any Georgia facility would really accept a critically ill patient on a ventilator, especially during the Covid crisis.

With the coronavirus numbers ramping up every day, ventilators were hard to come by, and most facilities were not accepting new patients due to concerns about contamination from the virus.

These are very difficult situations even in normal times. It is all too common for hospitals to do all they can to discharge patients who are dying, just so they can keep their statistics up and their risks down.

Based on Valerie's assessment of this client's dire condition, I shut down any attempt to discharge him from the hospital on the grounds that his life would be endangered if they tried to move him. There was no other safe place to transport him to at that point.

We had an emotional Zoom meeting with the patient's wife and three grown children.

Valerie described to them the failing condition of his lungs and heart and other major organs.

"I'm losing him, aren't I?" his wife asked me.

"Yes, I'm afraid you are," I said.

"Why didn't the hospital tell me this?" she asked.

It was a question I couldn't answer, even though I had my suspicions. This happens all too often with clients who are in the fragile years, hospitalized due to a stroke or a heart attack and no longer responsive. Family members are left in the dark and not given the information they need to make critical decisions.

I think that is unfair and cruel, and I always do my best to give them the truth so they can decide what to do. There were tears this time, from all of us, as the reality set in. The client's children were stunned because they had no idea of his condition until that point, but all of the family also expressed gratitude for our advocacy and efforts on behalf of their loved one.

His wife kept saying, "I'm so grateful for the truth; I feel calmer now than when I did not know."

Our next step was to determine where the family wanted him to be in his final hours.

"Home with me and the kids," his wife said.

We arranged to have him discharged from the hospital and taken home where we'd set up hospice care. He died thirty-six hours after coming home, with his loved ones present.

His widow called a few days later and expressed her gratitude for our assistance.

"I am at peace," she said. "I am sad that he is gone, but I am at peace."

As it turned out, this was a relatively easy case in the time of coronavirus. We had many more complex situations, including one in which a client who'd been taking care of his wife with Alzheimer's in their home could no longer handle it because she'd become combative and resistant to his efforts.

He could no longer handle her care on his own. He wanted to move her to an assisted living facility in Colorado that had a special unit for patients with her condition. They had accepted her earlier in the year but, at that point, the husband had not been ready to let her go.

The couple had a daughter who lived nearby, and she could provide support from there.

That plan fell through when the pandemic hit because the Colorado facility shut down new admissions. The husband's plan B was to move her into a local facility, but none of them were taking patients either because of the coronavirus threat.

We provided in-home caregivers to help the husband while we worked on this challenging case, but the professionals had their hands full with the woman. They were getting beat up as they tried to get her properly medicated without overmedicating her.

Our team spent hours on the telephone and finally convinced the assisted living facility in Colorado to take her as they had promised before the pandemic. She had already been approved, so they agreed to make an exception for her.

The challenge then was to find a way to transport the agitated Alzheimer's patient from Florida to Colorado. To our surprise, a kind neighbor, an angel really, agreed to drive her there. That is a true friend!

I share these stories with you now to give you an understanding of the challenges we face in the trenches day in and day out, in good times and in bad, as we advocate and assist clients in the fragile years. Mostly, I have written this book to give you hope and a realistic perspective by providing the information you need to make difficult decisions about your loved ones.

In some ways, my staff and I had it pretty easy during the first wave of the pandemic. None of our eighty clients in care facilities or under home care by our staff contracted the coronavirus, which is remarkable. It helped that the facilities we work with in Florida shut down early and took the threat very seriously.

My counterparts in other areas of the country had a much harder time because the pandemic hit them earlier and harder.

Geriatric Genocide

My friend Trish Colucci Barbosa, a registered nurse who served with me on the national board of the Aging Life Care Association, runs a Care Management company for older adults and clients with special needs in New Jersey. Her business is similar to my own in Central Florida.

In the spring of 2020, the coronavirus hit her state's nursing homes and other care facilities with such deadly force that some described it as "geriatric genocide."

"We had nine clients die in the first two or three weeks," Trish told me in anguish. "It was brutal on all of us. These were people we loved."

The first client she lost died within two days of being diagnosed, triggering alarms that sent Trish and her eight-member staff scrambling to check on their clients in nursing homes, home care, and hospitals.

"When people began falling like dominos, dying one after the other, we had a Zoom meeting where my staff and I just cried and shared our feelings," she said.

One of the hardest things was that neither their family members nor the eight members of Trish's staff could be with clients stricken by the contagious and deadly virus, she said.

"Nobody could get in to see them. We couldn't be at their bedsides to hold their hands," she recalled. "They all died alone."

Nearly 43 percent of those in the United States who died in the first wave of Covid-19 were residents in long-term care facilities, and those in New Jersey were particularly hard hit. Media reports said that 5,368 long-term care residents died in the state, roughly one in every thirteen residents.

Trish and her team kept fighting for their clients during the crisis, doing their best to keep those who were isolated in communication with concerned loved ones while also handling one emergency after another.

Like so many health care professionals on the front lines against the Covid-19 pandemic, they struggled with the unpredictable and highly contagious virus, its wide range of symptoms, and its resistance to the usual treatments. Some patients who appeared to be doing well died within days. Others who seemed on death's door recovered.

"People we thought would die didn't, and people we thought would make it didn't," Trish said. "We had a ninety-one-year-old client with a high fever who tested positive in May, and the doctors gave her only thirty-six hours. Her lips were blue at one point. We put her on hospice care, and she was getting morphine, but now she is fighting back, and I think she is going to survive. That is amazing, and just another example of how unpredictable this virus is."

In other cases, Trish said clients without respiratory issues who appeared to be holding their own with the virus would suddenly stop eating and go into rapid decline.

"We'd put them on IV fluids, but they seemed to just give up and die," she said. "There is just so much we still don't know about this virus."

Circling the Wagons

The Covid-19 crisis has convinced me that this book is needed now, more than ever. I began writing it before the pandemic turned homes for the aging into some of the most dangerous and embattled places on earth. During the quarantine, our jobs have become all the more important and all the more challenging.

Yet, our experiences during this unprecedented global pandemic made me even more dedicated to completing this book and getting it into the hands of families and their loved ones searching frantically for answers.

The guidance provided in *The Fragile Years* is not theoretical. It is hard-earned and proven. The case studies are true, drawn from our client files. In this book, I provide practical information and insights based on my forty years of experience in this field.

My staff and I are elder care veterans, champions of older adults and their staunch advocates. We have assisted more than twenty thousand men and women in navigating the often-bewildering maze of nursing homes, assisted living centers, hospices, hospitals, Medicare, Medicaid, VA benefits, pharmacies, and home health care services.

Our mission, always, is to protect the wishes and best interests of our clients and their loved ones, which can put us at loggerheads with medical professionals, insurers, the Veteran's Administration, and nursing home administrators. We are not intimidated, and we don't back down in protecting the most vulnerable members of our society.

I am the former national president of The Aging Life Care Association. I have a master's degree in public health administration and a master's certificate in gerontology. I have worked in this industry for forty years. I have been an administrator in continuing care retirement communities, which care for independent residents, as well assisted living and skilled nursing residents.

In 2019, I sold The Cameron Group to Arosa, a premier provider of integrated care management and caregiving services.

I connected with the owners based on our shared values, so I agreed to join their rapidly-growing company as Director of Care Management. In that position, I oversee training of care managers companywide. In addition, I continue to work with my clients, which is my passion. One of our primary goals is to attract and retain great caregivers, which helps us provide a high level of care for older adults.

My team and I are still in the field every day, working on behalf of clients and their families, helping them find safe lodging and the best available medical care, tracking down doctors, talking with insurers, and sorting out prescription meds. We strive to provide our fragile clients with the quality of life they desire and deserve in the final stages of their lives.

The Move to Greater Dependence

Every individual ages differently, but typically, we enter our most fragile years in our eighties. The fragile years are marked by greater difficulty in carrying on daily activities. The aging person in this stage may need a caregiver or at least someone to keep a close watch. Often, there is a life-altering "event" of some kind, such as a fall causing minor or serious injuries, an illness that requires hospitalization or surgery, a diminished memory, or impaired mental capacity.

While most of us know our parents will eventually enter this natural stage of late life, few are fully prepared for the challenges it brings. The purpose of this book is to prepare the loved ones and the aging parents for the fragile years so that they can deal with those challenges and, hopefully, maintain a comfortable quality of life.

Each chapter of the book includes a section called "Your Takeaway Tips" that offers my guidance as a veteran administrator and advocate in this field. I tell our clients that the complexities can be daunting, but a mastery of the laws, rules, and regulations—and very specific terminology—can empower them and their loved ones as they seek the best possible care.

This book provides the loved ones of aging men and women with the knowledge, language, information, resources, and emotional support they need when their mothers and fathers, aunts and uncles, or close friends enter their most fragile years.

My client Nancy's mother offers a typical example of an older person whose independent lifestyle and security is suddenly threatened. Nancy's mom had done well through her mid-eighties, living at home with her husband, socializing with friends, and seemed to be aging quite gracefully. Then, as happens so often, she had "an event" that put her in the fragile zone at the age of eighty-nine.

She began having memory issues and behaving erratically. At first, her husband adjusted and took care of her, but he soon became overwhelmed and unable to give her the attention she required in her confused state. She ended up in the hospital where she was put on a feeding tube and then discharged to a nursing home.

Nancy struggled with the fact that her mother could no longer live at home, but she could see that the responsibility of caring for her was also affecting her father's health and well-being. She hoped her mom would settle into the nursing home.

Instead, her mother rebelled. She did not like the feeding tube, nor did she like anyone helping her bathe. She was confused and angry, and she made it clear that she was "sick of living in a goddamn hospital" even though she was in a nursing home.

After Nancy's call, I made several visits to her mother in the nursing home to assess her temperament, medical condition, and environment. Her mom was combative at first, demanding to know who I was and what I was doing there. I explained that I was a social worker, and Nancy had asked me to help figure out why she was unhappy.

"I hate it here, get me out of here," she snapped.

She had a glint in her eye and a bristly personality, but she could also be quite funny. I always enjoy elderly clients with sharp edges. They keep things lively. She certainly had the nursing home staff on their toes, berating them at every opportunity.

I've spent all of my career working in that environment in various capacities. I understand the many challenges and heavy regulations they deal with. Nancy's mom was in a good nursing home, but it just wasn't the right place for her.

This nursing home had a low tolerance for high maintenance residents. They'd decided she was a risk for aspirating her food, so they'd put her on a diet of mostly pureed food to supplement her feeding tube.

It is difficult to move residents on feeding tubes into assisted living centers. They aren't allowed by state regulation.

I found a solution to this dilemma as Nancy and I were discussing her mother's situation. The daughter mentioned a story about her mother I'd never heard.

"One of mom's friends from church visited her a while back and brought her a couple of those tiny little hamburger sliders that she loves. She gobbled them right down, no problem."

So, there we had it. She didn't need the tube, so we could get her into assisted living if we removed it. Her mom could eat on her own. She just didn't like the thick, pureed meals that the nursing home had given her.

I spoke with the nursing home's doctor to remove the feeding tube. I prepared Nancy by telling her the doctor might resist, which often makes the children of elderly residents feel guilty and scared.

As expected, the nursing home's doctor refused to remove the feeding tube. He argued that she was at risk for aspirating, and she'd been losing weight because she wouldn't eat.

Nancy, who worked for a prominent law firm as a paralegal, had to remind him that she had power of attorney for her mother who had entrusted her to advocate for her. When the doctor still refused to remove the feeding tube, Nancy and I set up an appointment with their family doctor and had him remove it.

We then had her mother transferred into an assisted living home just a few blocks from Nancy's home. There, the mother had her own studio apartment in a special unit for the memory impaired. I can't say that she lived happily ever-after because that wasn't her personality, but she never demanded to move out. She lived comfortably for another three years before she died at the age of ninety-two.

She had a quality of life in those final years that was much more to her liking. Nancy gave her mother that gift, and I was grateful for the opportunity to help.

Most adult children are poorly prepared for the life-changing events that send their once-independent parents and loved ones into the fragile zone. Clients who find themselves suddenly dealing with the decline of an older person compare it to falling into an abyss.

They often have to make a series of heart-wrenching decisions in a high stress, alien environment with its own language, complex rules, and potentially devastating costs.

With little or no preparation, they have to figure out what is best for their parents in discussions with hospital administrators, physicians, medical insurance providers, nursing homes and assisted living centers, pharmacists, and caregivers.

Frustrations and guilt run high. Emotions run up against financial realities. Many feel they have to do whatever they can to get their loved one back to normal or healthy again—and that often is just not possible for those who've become so fragile at an advanced age.

Most people past the age of eighty cannot tolerate even minor surgeries without it seriously compromising their ability to function—walk, eat, and sleep, let alone go through rehabilitation. Most do not want to spend their remaining time being poked, prodded, plugged into machines, and kept awake in a hospital environment. Many complain about spending so much time at the doctors. I've even heard some say it's like a full-time job.

As a professional care manager and advocate for the aging, I am dedicated to pursuing compassionate strategies that follow the wishes of my fragile clients, who need to be protected and spared from well-intentioned but unnecessary procedures. I've written this book to help others serve as more effective advocates on behalf of aging loved ones.

After working in nursing home administration, I wanted to help aging people more directly, so I started my own business providing a full range of services. I struggled financially to launch my start-up, but our biggest problem once we were established was growing fast enough to meet the demand.

There was such a need for information in the early years that I couldn't hire fast enough. I heard over and over, "How do people find you? How do people navigate this without help?"

I didn't have even a website until 2006; I barely advertised. Most of my new clients learned of me from friends, family members, and neighbors.

My Mission

The Fragile Years is written for the 34.2 million unpaid caregivers and adult children of aging parents entering their final years of life. In 2012, the Baby Boomers began turning sixty-five, and their numbers now exceed more than seventy-five million. Ten thousand Baby Boomers turn sixty-five every day. This aging population has created a huge demand for helpful elder care information.

As they enter their most vulnerable stage of life, these seventy-five million Baby Boomers will rely mostly on their adult children and other family and friends to oversee their finances, medical treatments, prescriptions, health insurance, nursing home, assisted living, and hospice care—and hopefully other more creative options for staying at home in addition to palliative care options.

This book is a comprehensive how-to guide for those who will be squeezed for time and resources as they raise their own children and assist their aging parents while also holding down day jobs.

The Fragile Years speaks directly to these inexperienced, overwhelmed, and unpaid caregivers. In these pages, I provide the tools and information those with fragile parents—and all others who may be responsible for older loved ones—need to be prepared and to serve as compassionate, caring, and wise advocates themselves.

The information in this book will help loved ones make informed and compassionate decisions on these critical topics as well as many others. In addition, this guide should give caregivers confidence to make decisions that may appear contrary to the medical profession's opinions.

Among the areas of concern addressed are:

- *Preparing family members to serve as advocates for their aging parents before and after they become fragile*
- *Strategies for protecting the best interests and expressed desires of your loved one*
- *Recognizing your parent's entry into the fragile years*
- *Avoiding repeated hospitalizations and unnecessary treatments and surgeries*
- *Choosing the right place of care for your parent*
- *Recruiting quality caregivers with creative approaches*
- *Dealing with the special challenges of the memory-impaired parent*
- *Navigating the insurance maze, including Medicare, Medicaid, and VA benefits*

- *Understanding prescriptions, drug interactions, and mastering strategies to reduce medications*
- *Financial strategies for providing elder care without exhausting savings*

A Manifesto on Care for the Aging

Finally, this book is my labor of love for my clients, and my oldest and wisest friends and family members. It is also my manifesto, a call for a different level of care—a more compassionate approach based on the concept that for aging people, sometimes medical procedures like major surgery can cause more harm than benefit. I will encourage nursing homes and other care facilities to put the patient's desires first, and to allow them a more natural and peaceful end of life if that is what they desire.

As an expert in aging life care, I have marched in and demanded the release of hospitalized clients scheduled for unnecessary and potentially lethal surgeries. In the early days of my business, I sometimes even provided temporary lodging for clients in my own home, until my husband said it is one thing to bring my work home, another to bring nonagenarians and their incontinent pets.

I am cordial and professional in negotiating on behalf of my clients, yet I am always willing to challenge physicians, surgeons, hospital administrators, nursing home staff, and insurance-crats. I have stalked the halls of the US Veterans Administration lobbying for wiser policies, and I have testified before legislators on many of the topics covered in this book.

The business model that physicians and health care workers work within is a capitalized system designed to generate revenue and reduce the risk of lawsuits. While there are many great medical providers with big hearts who try to do the right thing, most know that the system is rigged.

Their goal is to bring profits up and costs down for the stakeholders, including hospitals, insurance and pharmaceutical companies, and nursing homes. This transactional approach collides with the desires of most aging adults who do not want to be subjected to batteries of tests and life-prolonging procedures.

I can be fierce in my advocacy, but my goal is always to provide those fragile clients under my care with an environment that follows their vision—one that is as pleasant, spiritual, and stress-free as possible. One that hopefully is marked by love, laughter, and gratitude.

With this book, I hope to serve as a lightning rod for change. We need to focus on providing better and more thoughtful care for our most vulnerable citizens, aging men and women. I want to inspire politicians, business leaders, and health care professionals to do better for our older loved ones.

One day, we will all reach the final stages of our lives, our most fragile years, and each of us will want to know that someone is looking out for us.

Chapter Two

Recognizing Your Loved One's
Entry into the Fragile Years

Late in his life, my father took to calling me, "Four."
I was born the fourth of six children, and I guess this was his way of keeping track of all of us and where we fit in the family lineup.

"Hey Four!" he'd say when we talked on the phone or saw each other for the first time in a while.

I didn't mind, but I did prefer the other nickname he gave me later on whenever I helped him pay his bills and balance his checkbooks. He only came to me for help with that once his mental abilities began to diminish. He'd tell me, "We need to have a meeting."

At these monthly meetings, he would first try to do all the calculating, but eventually he'd just hand it over to me and let me figure it out. That's when he called me by my other nickname, "Brilliant."

"You really are brilliant, you know," he'd say when I finished his paperwork, which wasn't all that complicated.

I loved being there for my father in his fragile years. I felt empowered as I helped him, using all the expertise I'd built up as a professional in the field of aging care management. And I have to say, my father's life ended in probably the best way possible, if there is such a thing.

His decline was gradual and without any catastrophic events causing him pain and suffering. I was with him when he died. He took his last breath with my husband and me at his bedside in a rural Michigan nursing home. It was run by a kind country doctor who provided palliative care (pain management) to my father and all the residents in two nursing homes across the road from each other.

Dad knew we were there. I did my best to calm him and ease his mind.

It was very emotional, yet also moving and beautiful to be there and let him know that he was loved. I'd been preparing for that moment while watching my father become increasingly fragile in the preceding years, but I was overcome with grief nonetheless. That is only natural, of course, and part of loving and being loved.

Although I knew he had entered the fragile years and was on his last leg of life, it didn't make it easier to watch him decline. Nor did my expertise give me full immunity to the denial that adult children often experience when they see their aging parents slipping. Their mortality reminds us of our own. Too often, we refuse to admit we might be losing them and, as a result, we aren't properly prepared to step in as they become more dependent and vulnerable.

Many adult children don't notice a parent's initial entry into the fragile years until there is a big wake-up call, like a heart attack, or smaller signs such as unpaid bills piling up. Later, family members may recall other indications of decline that they failed to notice.

In my conception of The Fragile Years™, there are five steps or stages recognized as indicators of decline in an aging person. By defining this time of life, my goal is to help ensure the wishes of older loved ones are honored when it comes to the care they receive—or do not receive—at this stage.

This concept has helped many family members accept that their parents should not undergo major surgeries or extensive rehabilitation plans that might end their days more quickly or greatly diminish their quality of life in their final stages.

Stage One: A reduction in the number of times per week they participate in their favorite social activities like golf, lunches with friends, volunteering/working, and church and club meetings.

Stage Two: Losing interest in activities outside the home. They may say they don't have the energy anymore; or maybe they only go if someone offers to take them or nudges them.

Stage Three: The parent just wants to stay home and may no longer do minor chores like taking out the garbage or retrieving the mail or newspapers. They may skip meals unless someone else prepares them or nap more often. At this stage some may say it takes "too much energy to live." You might also notice a loss of interest in their family members and their activities.

Stage Four: The parent rarely leaves a favorite chair or bed as movement even within the residence is cut way back. When the elder does move about, it may be just from one resting place to another, with slow progress.

Stage Five: The parent sleeps and naps most of the day. Eats very little. Drinks little. Speech and mobility slow to a crawl.

The First Stage: Pulling Back

My late father's gradual shift from an active life into the fragile years followed the classic stages, and I share his story with you to provide insights that could be helpful with your own loved ones one day. He was married, and I am one of six children, so this story will be told through my eyes and perceptions.

Dad was always a very active guy. A tool and die maker by trade, he moved into sales and then into the ranks of management, rising to become president of a steel foundry. He loved to socialize and to tinker in his workshop or on household projects.

Initially, he did not slow down much at all in retirement. My father and stepmother actually worked at a resort in Wyoming one summer. They traveled often, sightseeing and visiting family. He played golf as often as seven times a week. In his "retirement," he also started several businesses, worked at a local golf course, and spent many hours making beautiful tables and credenzas in his well-equipped wood-working shop on their farm. Dad's fifteen minutes of fame came when a local newspaper reported that he could "golf his age" in his early eighties.

A few years into his retirement, he began to pull back on some of his activities, but just a little at first. We all noticed when he curtailed his golfing to just a couple times a week. On his second trip to spend part of the winter in Florida with me, he didn't golf at all. That's when it really hit me.

The second event came when he stopped driving and turned over his car keys. "I scared myself," he said, while declining to elaborate. After that, he had to be driven to lunch to see his friends at the local Bob Evans restaurant. Then he lost all interest in meeting up with them.

The first step into the fragile years usually occurs when our aging loved ones are in their mid to late eighties. I should note that there are always many exceptions to this, including many genetically blessed people who are still walking mountain trails in their nineties.

We may fail to notice as they gradually move to a slower pace, tighten their social circles, and cut back on excursions and outings for favorite activities.

Another indicator that my father wanted to slow down was the fact that he declined an invitation to his granddaughter's college graduation at Carnegie Mellon University in Pennsylvania. Just four years earlier, he'd been enthusiastic in celebrating her high school graduation. Dad had even walked across the football stadium field to congratulate her, though he needed help getting back to his seat.

On this visit, he napped every day at 3 p.m., no matter what other plans we might present. He also liked to "rest my eyes for a while" in bed in the mid-morning on days when he was up early.

These were all indications that my father was entering the first stage of his fragile years. By the time my father hit eighty-four, he had been diagnosed with frontotemporal dementia. His mind was not as quick, and his pace was slowing. His neuropathy, causing numbness in his feet, had advanced and, like many of his age, he had no patience or interest in working with a physical therapist for rehabilitation.

This is very common as older people enter the fragile years. They may see a physical therapist, but they are not interested in doing the exercises at home. The stretching and bending can be painful for them, and at this stage in life, they don't see that there will be any long-term rewards, or they don't care about long-term rewards.

My clients in this stage have told their children things like: "I'm not entering any more marathons, you know."

My sister and I were trying to get our father to use a cane, and his response was to create his own walking sticks. It was a bit of a cliff hanger watching him use those sticks, and eventually he did transition to the cane, but some support was better than none, so we went with it.

Dad took great pride in creating, building, and fixing things. His crafted canes proved to be good conversation starters on his strolls.

The Second Stage: Looking in the Rearview Mirror

A very common sign of this stage is a tendency toward nostalgia and reflection on life—a focus on their past instead of their future. One friend remembers realizing that his father had entered this stage when he requested a trip back to his boyhood hometown to view his childhood home, his high school, and favorite haunts.

"He didn't want to get out of the car, really," my friend recalled. "He just wanted to drive around and reminisce. He made me drive around his high school and his old neighborhood a couple times as he reflected on his years there."

During one of my visits to my father's home in Michigan, he asked me to take him for a drive to view the farms and countryside that he loved.

Giving up the wheel was a big thing for him, and one trip stands out for me as he had a very specific destination in mind.

"I want to take you to my favorite burger place," he said.

Dad gave me very specific directions, telling me every turn to make, but we couldn't find it. We drove around for hours, which was okay with me. The countryside was lovely, and I enjoyed having the one-on-one time to talk to him.

I had noticed his memory was not as sharp as it once had been, and after a couple hours of driving all over the area, I began to seriously wonder if he had any idea where this burger place was located.

Just as I became convinced we'd never find it, he told me to make another turn, and darned if it wasn't right there!

As I drove into the parking lot, he gave me a look I knew all too well. It was his "Never doubt your Dad" look. My doubts about the power of his memory might have been temporarily eased, though after we'd eaten, I did have some questions about his sense of taste.

The place had the *worst* hamburgers I'd ever eaten in my life!

But Dad was in heaven. He was so happy about sharing his favorite greasy spoon with me, and I was even more happy to be there with him.

I share this story with you because this is a common experience for those with aging parents at this stage as they enter their eighties.

Just when you think maybe it's time to have "the talk" about them moving in with you, or into a nursing home or similar facility, the parent will surprise you a moment later with some keen observation, sharp memory, or other display of competence.

So, what do we do as their children? Too often, we put off making plans with them or preparing ourselves for what is to come. The signs of declining abilities are often harder to spot for those loved ones who see the aging person every day. If you see them only sporadically, the changes are easier to pick up on.

This can create tensions between siblings or family members. Those who are with the parent every day may be more inclined to just leave them alone. Those who visit only occasionally may push for more aggressive actions. I've found that there are often differing opinions about the parent's needs between the local child and the long-distance child.

Families are often torn, and as a result they delay intervening, or suggesting medical or mental tests, or getting services in the home. Most of us want to honor our aging family members, respect their dignity, and let them remain independent and in control as long as they can.

Our parents also may well assert their independence and try to hang on to their dignity and autonomy, even when they aren't as mobile or sharp-minded as they once were. Just when we want to intercede, they can surprise us with flashes of insight and pride.

One day, I took my father shopping for a new recliner chair. One of my pet peeves is that they don't design good looking furniture with aging customers in mind. Most are too deep and wide. (I may one day design my own brand of couches and reading chairs with easy ingress and egress for older folks. But, I digress.)

We went to at least six stores trying to find a well-built chair that he could get in and out of easily. Dad was weary by the time we hit the last store. He was using his walker and moving slowly through the showroom when he approached a group of men blocking his path.

They looked to be corporate guys from the headquarters of this big chain of furniture stores. Intent on their discussion, none of them even looked up as he walked toward them.

Dad sensed that they didn't think this "old guy" was worthy of the slightest acknowledgement by these "young bucks."

I could tell that my father was irritated by their lack of respect. After all, he was once a corporate executive himself. He shot me a look as if to say, "I've got this."

Then he waded into them, brandishing his cane and saying loudly, "Man coming through!"

The guys in suits backed off. My father was delivering a message, one that many older people would agree with. He was saying, "I'm old, but I'm not invisible. I am still a human being worthy of notice."

The Third Stage: Giving Up Independence

My dad's chronic complaint was that his legs didn't work right, and he was convinced there was a cure for them. When his cardiologist recommended he have heart valve surgery, my father thought that would cure his leg pains. My nurse sister couldn't convince him otherwise.

Dad took it to heart when his cardiologist said, "If you don't have this surgery, you will be dead in a year." I am not sure how this physician knew that. There are no studies to back it up. Nonetheless, much to the family's dismay, dad went into surgery.

Cardiologists and surgeons may refer to this as "routine surgery," but nothing is routine with patients in their eighties. I know this from my experiences with clients, but at this point, Dad was still living independently, and it wasn't my call to make.

None of us fought him. I made my case against the surgery, and so did my father's long-time dermatologist who treated him for skin cancer.

"Your life will not be the same if you go through with this surgery," he told my father.

At one point, Dad had decided not to do it, but something changed his mind.

He went ahead and had the surgery, and afterwards, he was never as strong mentally or physically again. He had a vacant look that never really left him. It was sad because none of his mobility or stamina problems improved.

He also seemed to lose a lot of his spark. He had what is known as a "flat affect." He didn't express much emotion, either good or bad, and although he wasn't ever an emotional guy, he lost what little he had displayed in the past. This can be the result of depression, or stress, or a result of medications and anesthesia.

Shortly after his surgery, my father let us know he was ready for a change in his usual schedule. We were all surprised, but there was no changing his mind. He asked if he could come down to Florida in June instead of waiting until December. He was adamant. This time, he wanted to fly down rather than drive, which was a good decision.

We were worried about accommodating him since his wife didn't want to come. All of his friends and other family members were in Michigan, yet he was determined to fly down.

In our telephone discussions with Dad about making this major lifestyle change, I noticed that he sometimes seemed disoriented and had difficulty focusing on the conversations. I worried that he had made this strange decision because of some form of dementia. That thought also made me concerned about his ability to navigate the airport and baggage claim.

When I expressed some concern, my father insisted he wouldn't have any problems. So, I went along with his plan.

On the day of his arrival, I called my father as soon as his flight landed and told him I was inside the airport waiting for him. I tried to guide him to my location on the phone, but I could tell he was confused by the directions.

It quickly became apparent that he was having serious issues figuring out where he was. I called airport security to help locate him. Security tracked him down and brought him to me in a wheelchair. He seemed even more confused when I talked to him in person.

He was wearing his favorite hat and grinning from ear to ear. As I drove him home, he turned to me and said, "I think I might be having some memory problems."

My dad was a very proud man, a big, self-assured guy who'd done well as an executive in a tough business. Admitting that he felt vulnerable had to be difficult for him. He was circling the wagons. I felt a pressure with a layer of sadness unlike anything I had ever felt. He seemed even more confused in person than he had over the phone.

The Fourth Stage: Looking for a Soft Place to Land

My father moved into our condo near Orlando. My husband, Regan, and I had to go to work every day, but that seemed to be fine with him. He quickly settled into a routine. He'd have breakfast, then he'd take our dog, Stevie, for a walk, return around 11 a.m., and take a nap until lunchtime. After lunch, he and Stevie took another walk. They always went on the same route, but, as Dad would say, "Clockwise in the morning. Counterclockwise in the afternoon!"

After the late walk each day, Dad would sit outside near the lake or on our porch and read a book for an hour or two before his afternoon nap. There was no negotiating on his nap times. Any appointments or trips had to be scheduled around them.

When he arose from his afternoon nap, he'd then have dinner with us, finishing in time to settle in front of the television and watch *Wheel of Fortune* and then *Jeopardy*. Then it was lights out by 8 p.m. This was a very comfortable routine for everyone except for maybe Stevie. Our little ten-pound dog somehow gained three pounds while taking two walks a day and hanging out with my father.

Dad was always a fun-loving guy, the sort who would pretend to pull coins from children's ears. He still could turn on the charm when he had an audience, even in his later years. A natural storyteller, he kept us entertained with stories at mealtimes, though sometimes we had to wonder if he was making up some things. He talked about an "Aunt Maggie" that none of us had ever heard of.

I'd take him to lunch at work with my staff now and then, and he'd keep them enthralled with his tales. Dad was not as gregarious and on-the-go as he'd been in his sixties and early seventies but was still very sociable at this point. He was always a people-person who enjoyed engaging with everyone he encountered. Within a short time, everyone in our building and the neighborhood seemed to know him.

He was also quite popular at our local Publix, Lowe's, and Home Depot, where he'd ride around in the electric carts provided and chat up the other shoppers, shelf-stockers, butchers, and checkout staff. He enjoyed the mobility and freedom to wander at will while riding a cart. Sometimes, he actually put items in his cart basket, but mostly he served as an unofficial greeter and shopping advisor.

He seemed very happy, which is why we were surprised when just two months into staying with us, Dad asked me out of the blue: "Do you think I'd like living in one of those assisted living places where some of your clients live?" This almost *never* happens with an older adult, and I was really shocked when he brought it up.

I didn't try to talk him out of this move because I did think he might want to be around more people his age. His big question was whether he could afford assisted living. He showed me his bank account because although I helped him pay his bills, I had no idea how much money he'd saved for retirement.

His savings weren't really enough for a long-term facility, but again, my years of working with aging clients paid off with my father. As a Korean War vet, he was eligible for the VA's Aid and Attendance benefit.

Under this program, the VA will pay a monthly pension for qualified veterans and surviving spouses of wartime veterans for long-term care at home or in assisted living. They have to have served at least ninety days of active duty with at least one day during war time. I will explain this benefit in greater depth later in the book.

When the VA transferred the retroactive funds into his bank account, I handed him his bank statement. He looked at the recent deposit and said, "This is the strangest business deal I've ever been involved in. I didn't have to do a thing and money just magically appeared in my account."

The Fifth Stage: A Peaceful Passing

Dad seemed to settle into life at the assisted living home near our condo, so we were once again surprised when he announced after several months there that he wanted to return to his rural Michigan hometown. He and his wife missed each other, and the pull to return had to be honored.

My sister and stepmother found a place there, closer to his old friends and favorite haunts. He had just turned eighty-six years old. Again, I didn't try to discourage him, but I was sad to see him go so far away.

Selfishly, I wanted to keep him close, but my philosophy with my aging clients is always to allow them to choose the life they want, as long as they are still capable of making good decisions and financially able to do it. And so, at that late stage, he returned to the place where he'd spent most of his life. I certainly couldn't begrudge him that final move.

My sister Beth, the nurse, was also a fierce advocate for him. We worked with the staff at the care community to help them know and understand my father and his needs. I was able to make frequent visits to see him, and Beth kept all of us informed as to how he was doing. Family cooperation is essential in caring for a fragile parent. My sister was an ideal teammate.

After our father had been in the care community nearly six months, the staff reported that he seemed to be in decline.

"Your dad is eating less, and he seems to be slowing way down," they told me. He was having difficulty getting up and walking, which forced him to use his wheelchair more. The final action that required his move to a nursing home was his inability to get in and out of bed without assistance.

My sister found a rural nursing home that had a bed available, and he was transferred there with no problems. Beth and my father's wife realized that he was nearing life's end. We needed to adjust his care to allow him a natural and peaceful death.

"He needs palliative care, which would help him die peacefully and without pain," the doctor said. "We can provide that for him here."

I observed this doctor take wonderful care of my dad, giving him just the right amount of medication, activity, and attention. At least one family member saw Dad nearly every day.

On my second to last visit to the nursing home, I could see the end coming for my father. He'd always been a man of routine. He rarely changed his breakfast, for example, always having a cup of coffee, a cup of hot chocolate, and his favorite Egg McMuffin from McDonald's.

One of my favorite memories is of making my version of Egg McMuffins for him every morning, but I suspected he liked the McDonald's version more. When I visited him on this trip, Dad was still clinging to his routine, but he had slowed way down.

I drove to McDonald's to get his breakfast and brought it back to the nursing home. I watched him lift the hot chocolate to his mouth, and at one point he was holding it in midair. Then he put a straw in it, gave up, and stared into space.

He was dying, but in a good place, surrounded by family, and attended to by a terrific medical team offering hospice-quality care in the nursing home. In the days that followed, my father no longer wanted to sit up in a wheelchair. He preferred to remain in bed. When they sat him up to eat, he told them he was not hungry or thirsty.

In his last weeks, Dad spent many hours looking out his window at the rural landscape. He described to me what he saw in vivid detail. There were farm animals, but also buffalos and eagles, he said.

I didn't try to correct him or challenge him. His visions were part of his rite of passage, and our discussions were profound in those final days. My father had been a world traveler, and he'd come home to die in peace.

I was grateful for the time we'd had to reconnect and to prepare our goodbyes. As I noted earlier, his passing was about as good as any of us could hope for.

A Major Event

In the late stages of the fragile years, there is often an event that accelerates a decline in health or mental acuity. Often it is a fall, a stroke or series of strokes, or a heart attack. The adult children will get the dreaded phone call from a caregiver, a nurse, or a family member: "Your mom is in the hospital."

In many cases, this is when services like mine are called in, although we recommend, and wish, that we become involved sooner because there is no soft-pedaling that tough decisions must be made and made quickly.

In Dad's case, he'd had heart valve replacement surgery three years earlier, and though it had set him back, he was still able to enjoy life for another three years or so. Often, the person doesn't have that much time to say goodbye.

The fragile years are marked by heightening concerns and emotions. The aging parent and the person's loved ones are all vulnerable. Their hearts tell them one thing while their doctors and other health care providers may tell them something entirely different.

Life becomes much more complex as loved ones are drawn into the unfamiliar and complicated world of hospitals, surgeons, medical insurance, nursing homes, assisted living centers, memory impairment programs, and home care. They often receive conflicting advice from these sources. Often, loved ones feel that they've entered an alien universe where a different language is spoken.

That is why I believe it is wise to be prepared on many levels for an aging family member to enter the fragile years. In most cases, family members and loved ones know that the time is running short, but they are hesitant to take action because they don't want to upset the aging parent or face the reality themselves, and they don't realize that help is available to them.

These are the most common mistakes we make as caregivers for our older loved ones:

- Failing to recognize that the aging person has become more and more fragile and far less independent.
- Becoming over-controlling and not considerate of their wishes.
- Because of our own anxiety about their fragility, we make decisions based on our own emotions rather than being more thoughtful and exploring options.
- Not understanding the risks of leaving a fragile person unattended.

- Refusing to work with them to put their needs first. There are many gray areas that the loved ones have to deal with. If a fragile parent is determined to remain independent and in their home, you can avoid upsetting them by providing part-time "housekeepers" who are really experienced aides, or you can send a pizza over so they don't have to cook on a weekend. Gradual change works better than forcing some big change on them.

- Misjudging the level of their mental impairment. Often, the fragile older person may think they are doing fine or want to believe they are doing fine; but if they are in danger or putting others in danger, the loved ones have to make difficult decisions.

- Neglecting to check in on them regularly with face-to-face meetings online or visits in person. In many cases, we've had loved ones discover stacks of unpaid bills or decaying food left out by an aging person who has experienced a sudden and rapid decline in judgement.

- Taking on guardianship without understanding the full responsibilities and what that entails.

- Not fully grasping the physical challenges faced by the aging person. I had a client who insisted that her mother go to an exercise class when the poor woman had a spinal condition that made it agonizing for her.

- Adopting the attitude that your roles have reversed, and you are now parent and your parent is the child. This is a dangerous position to take, and often the aging person will find it repugnant and rebel against it. It is advisable to approach them as a partner and to work with them rather than telling them what to do.

Your Takeaway Tips:

- *I knew of an elderly gentleman who carried his checkbook with him to pay off the owners of cars that he hit while driving each day. He racked up thousands in damage payments. Check your aging parent's car for dents and other damage to ascertain if the time has come to limit or stop them from driving.*

- *Visit or have someone check in on your parent regularly to monitor for changes in daily routines, behaviors, moods, and personal hygiene.*

- *Install a motion detector security camera to alert you to changes in routine and possible emergencies.*

- *Be very observant and note when your parent stops once-favorite activities.*

- *Make note of how fast your parent is moving. One case study showed that the slowing pace of an older person serves as a predictor of life expectancy.*

- *Stay with your parents a couple times a year for seventy-two hours to just be with them. There is no better way to really see and feel how your parents are doing than staying with them.*

- *It can be helpful to tell them how much it means to be returning the love and care they gave you. If the loved one wasn't there for you, one option is to tell the person that it would help you if they sought assistance because you are worried about them.*

- *Sometimes there is nothing that can be done until an "event," in which case be ready with a plan when the crisis finally does occur.*

Chapter Three

Preparing for Your Parent's Fragile Years

Don and June had each been married previously and both had grown-up children. They were single when they met in their late eighties. They married after a brief courtship. They'd been married just three years when they both entered their fragile years.

That's when things got complicated, as they often do. Don and June were living together in their home when their loved ones became concerned about their ability to take care of themselves.

June's adult children wanted the couple to move into an assisted living center. Don's children thought they were okay staying in their home if home care assistance was provided.

Even Don and June were not clear on where they should live. One wanted to stay at home. The other claimed to have no preference.

There were multiple family members with power of attorney and multiple health care surrogates brought in. Some legal documents allowed the parents to make their own decisions. Others put the children in charge.

My team was called in by one of several lawyers involved. We provided home health care and made sure Don and June had safe living conditions and that their health was monitored. We stabilized the situation and managed their home care.

But there was an ongoing tug of war over who had the right to make decisions for the couple, as well as what those decisions should be. There was also a concern that the person in charge of making health care decisions shouldn't be managing Don and June's money matters.

One solution would be to go to a court-appointed guardian, but this was not a wealthy family. There would be substantial legal fees added to all of the other costs they were incurring at this critical point in their lives. Our team tried to act as impartial arbitrators in this situation. There were no good guys and bad guys. Everyone was trying to do what they thought was best for their loved ones.

Now, this may seem like a worst-case scenario, and it is certainly complex, but it is not all that uncommon. Their story illustrates a point that I often raise when speaking to siblings with concerns about an aging parent or other family member: having all their personal paperwork in order and having a clear plan in place for your parents and loved ones can save everyone involved from a lot of stress.

I've seen siblings and entire families torn apart because of their conflicting views on what an aging loved one wants or needs after a life-changing event that makes the older person dependent on them. If there is already disharmony and dysfunction in a family, a loved one's sudden decline will put even more strain on the relationships.

There are three key areas to focus on in making preparations for your parent's fragile years.

1. Strengthening family bonds and creating a plan of action.
2. Determining the aging loved one's preferences for their final years.
3. Locating, organizing, and updating the aging person's personal paperwork, including all legal, medical, and financial records and contacts.

Strengthening Family Bonds

Julia called me with concerns about her aging mother, who was living with her brother. Julia was worried that her brother was not providing adequate care for their mother.

"I will visit her and do a wellness check for you," I told her, "but my evaluation will be based on what I find, whether or not it confirms your suspicions about your brother's fitness as a caretaker."

She agreed to my ground rules, and as it turned out, I found that the brother was providing good care for their mother. Julia accepted my findings and then we worked on creating a plan for the mother's care while building trust between the two siblings she relied on. When there are deeply-entrenched issues, you might consider family counseling so that lingering resentments and anger do not get in the way of your parent's care in the final stages of life. This can save many years of guilt and grief. In my experience, those who grieve the passing of a parent the most are the family members who never resolved their conflicts with the loved one.

Most of us tend to avoid emotionally-wrenching discussions, especially as our parents become more fragile. We think, "I'll bring this up another time." Too often, though, time runs out, and the healing we want never comes. I'm not a grief counselor, but from personal and professional experience, I know there is healing to be found in forgiveness.

Sadly, an aging parent's entry into the fragile years often begins with a crisis, whether it's an injury from a fall, a stroke, a heart issue, or a sudden decline in mental acuity. Your loved one will need unified and organized support. If there are unresolved, long-standing conflicts between family members, chaos can ensue when you most need a unified front and a well-organized plan of action.

The most common issues I've seen cause family tension when a parent turns fragile are:

- Conflicting views over a course of action
- How much care will cost, and either the parent or one of the siblings can't agree about the costs
- Understanding the loved one's medical, mental, and emotional challenges
- Determining the level and type of care needed and where it should be provided (move to another facility or in-home care?)
- Finding a comfortable and safe place for the loved one to live
- The daunting task of collecting, organizing, and updating the paperwork on health insurance, prescriptions, Social Security, veteran's benefits, pensions, financial records, mortgages, utilities, and other bills

Practical Approaches

There are a few practical and proactive things you and your family members can do in planning for your loved one's fragile years.

Hopefully your parents have communicated who they want to be their power of attorney. If they haven't chosen someone, I suggested that a family member gently bring up the topic by saying something like this: "In case there is a crisis, we want to know who is assigned to legally represent you and follow your wishes."

If the individual can't leave home, many attorneys will make house calls. If this seems impossible to broach with them, hire a care manager or another trusted advisor to have this discussion. It's amazing how much work can get done when the person managing the work is not a relative!

You certainly should talk through possible scenarios as a family to make sure you are all on the same page, and then give the appointed decision maker your support. This trusted family member can take the point in dealing with doctors, nursing home administrators, lawyers, financial advisors, and all other critical contacts when fast action is required.

However, you might want to consider dividing up some of the responsibilities as far as family communications, bill-paying, investment monitoring, regular medical care, transportation, and other needs. So many times, the bulk of these responsibilities fall in the lap of the family member or members who live in closest proximity to the fragile loved one, but that doesn't have to be the case.

Many tasks can now be performed and monitored long distance thanks to the internet, apps, and video conferencing tools like Zoom, Houseparty, FaceTime, and others. So, help each other out as you work to help out your aging loved one. And if there is one family member who is shouldering more than others, consider setting up a schedule where others provide that person with occasional or regular support and relief, including filling in while they take vacations or days off.

You might even consider providing financial compensation to one family member so that person can cut back to a part-time job to devote more attention to the loved one.

Another practical thing to do, which may seem obvious but is often overlooked, would be to compile a comprehensive contact list for all family and friends of the aging individual.

Often we assume we have that information "somewhere," but making up and distributing a list of phone numbers, email addresses, and home addresses to assure quick and effective communication can be essential in emergencies. You also may want to organize a phone chain call system where, in an emergency, you can have calls made automatically to all essential contacts.

And last but not least, your family may be well-served by having calm and reasoned preliminary discussions about the eventual dispersal of family keepsakes, heirlooms, vacation and investment properties, and valuable art, jewelry, and vehicles. I know, you may cringe at the thought of even bringing up such topics. You don't have to make final decisions, but just knowing who would like to have what, or what the true value of certain items is can help you avoid conflict down the road when emotions are raw and everyone is grieving.

A Word of Caution about the "Role Reversal" Trap

I often cringe when I hear the adult children of fragile loved ones talk about how they feel like they've reversed roles with their parents who are now dependent on them. That attitude is a trap that can result in bitterness and resentment on both sides. Parents don't like their children telling them what to do—no matter how fragile they might be.

There is a much healthier way to engage with the new family dynamic, and that is to view this as an opportunity to become your parent's strongest advocate and supporter—a source of kindness, compassion, and understanding.

You aren't reversing roles. You are entering a new stage of your relationship. This isn't a burden; it's an opportunity to make your loved one's final years as comfortable, peaceful, and secure as possible.

Consider this also as your time to demonstrate to your own family, especially your children and grandchildren, how you would hope to be treated in the later stages of your own life. One of the keys to dealing with an aging parent is to let go of expectations that they will be fully capable of caring for themselves, or of conducting themselves perfectly or even up to your expectations.

For example, there may come a time when your loved one will turn inward and be much less communicative. Very often, the older adult is quieter, more introspective, and less interested in "making" conversation. This can make children and visitors very uncomfortable, so they try to "get" them to talk.

Consider that they might be in a stage or a phase where they are more introspective and processing information, memories, and reflecting. They might be uncomfortable out of fear of "being a burden" to the family. They might also feel guilty at how much you are doing for them.

Another consideration: you might not be asking the right questions and listening to their answers carefully. Be willing to ask questions with the intent of determining their state of mind as well as their wants and needs. Don't expect them to ask. They may be experiencing fear and insecurities about their own fragility and the approaching end of life.

Just knowing that you are there for them will be a great comfort. If you sense they are uncomfortable disclosing things to you, maybe there is a non-relative who can provide a valued, listening ear to them.

As an advocate for the aging, my priority is always the safety, comfort, and desires of the most fragile among us. I've learned to accept their quirks and often unpredictable behaviors, and I encourage their family members to do the same, rather than over-reacting when "Mom did something weird today."

I once had outraged members of a neighborhood watch committee demand that an elderly woman living in her own home be transferred against her will into an assisted living facility. They had called an adult protective services agency to investigate her behavior as a first step into removing her from their community.

The agency had contacted the woman's adult children, who lived in another state and were flipping out about the thought of their mother being forced out of her home. The children sent me to calm everyone down.

This woman was my client and I loved her. She'd been a stand-up comic in New York City for years and, despite some memory impairment, she was still hysterically funny at times.

She was doing quite well with assistance from a home care aide who came to help her each day. I couldn't imagine what she'd done to upset the neighborhood watch crew. I met with them to run interference for her when the agency informed me of their complaints.

"What's your issue with her?" I asked them.

"She goes to her mailbox every day in her see-through night-gown!" they complained.

Now, first of all, it was not see-through, just a nice light fabric, very chic and not at all tarty. But the neighbors were up in arms for some reason—as if a slightly eccentric elderly woman was a threat to their safety and home values?

I convinced my client to let her fully-clothed home care aide bring in the mail to keep the neighborhood alarmists from suffering trauma due to the sight of a graceful elderly woman checking the mailbox in her sleepwear.

This lack of understanding and intolerance of "senior moments" or eccentricities is distressing to me. What happened to the days when we welcomed neighbors like the fictional but legendary "Gladys Kravitz" who spied through her windows at her *Bewitched* neighbors in that television comedy series from the sixties and seventies?

I have seen the same lack of tolerance even in facilities that cater to older folks. I once had an assisted living facility administrator complain that my client who lived there was continually going off menu and off the grounds.

"He leaves every day to get a Big Mac at McDonald's!" came the complaint. We can't have him eating a hamburger every day!

Now, if this elderly man was suffering serious weight gain or loss because of his love of fast food, I might have been concerned, but he was doing just fine. He was relatively healthy and quite happy. So why not accommodate him in his fragile years?

"Maybe you should offer to make him your version of a Big Mac," was my suggestion. "If that makes him happy, why wouldn't you?"

In another case, I had a 102-year-old client who was labeled an escape risk by her assisted living administrator because she liked to take a walk in the parking lot to get some fresh air.

"We can't have her living here because she keeps escaping," the administrator said.

My client wasn't going anywhere. Even if she had wanted to flee, which she didn't, there was no way she could have made it out of the parking lot. The poor woman had extreme swelling in her legs and feet that made walking extremely difficult. She moved at a snail's pace and grew tired easily.

When your loved ones enter the fragile zone, they literally slow down. Their activity levels, their speech, the time it takes for them to dress, shower, and complete a meal—everything takes longer. I've heard it said that first marriage and then parenthood teaches us patience, and having a parent in the fragile years is yet another advanced lesson in the practice of that virtue.

Embrace it as part of life at this stage. The loved ones of aging people will find greater peace if they try to be more understanding, flexible, and accepting of their behavior—just as you would hope people will be when you enter this stage of life. Protect them from harm, certainly, but give them the freedom to fully enjoy themselves as long as no harm is done.

And be kind to yourselves and the others who love this person as well. You will very likely experience stress, anxiety, frustration, and even early grieving as your parent ages into the fragile zone. Understand that those are quite natural and almost universal feelings and also part of the human experience of loving and being loved.

I've seen far too many family members and friends feel like the aging of a parent is a burden or something that should be shouldered like a burden. If your fragile loved one depends on you at all, I encourage you to accept that responsibility as an act of love. And I suggest that you don't take this on without lightening your existing load as much as possible.

I say this from personal experience. I am one of those who tend to take on too many projects and responsibilities. When my father was living with us in his increasingly fragile years, I should have relinquished most of my other responsibilities so that I could have put more of my energy and time into him. I regret that.

Maybe you could step down temporarily from your extracurricular duties on boards, civic, or social groups so you can be there in your loved one's final years, months, or days. I promise you that you will not regret it.

Determine Your Loved One's Preferences

I've worked with many families overwhelmed by the complex and emotional decisions they face when a previously healthy and self-sufficient parent becomes dependent upon them. That is why I encourage you to prepare for a parent's fragile years by talking to them about their preferences for care.

Eighty percent of Americans say they would prefer to die at home, but only 20 percent are actually home when they die. Sixty percent die in acute care. Twenty percent die in nursing homes. Yet, in our experience, the best place for clients to spend their final hours is at home with loved ones.

I recommend having these discussions when your loved ones are still in good health and clear-minded, but I know that isn't always easy. If you can't get them to discuss their priorities and values regarding their later years of life, another option is to simply look at the decisions they've made over the years.

Have they been quick to go to the doctor or the hospital if they have a medical issue, or do they avoid seeking medical attention? A loved one who makes regular visits to the doctor would most likely want all possible measures taken to be kept alive if they have a heart attack, or stroke, or some other major medical challenge. But someone who has avoided medical care and hospitals would more likely not want extraordinary measures to be taken to prolong life if it meant long-term incapacitation or a severe decline in quality of life.

To find out what your parent wants, you don't have to pressure them. I had a friend whose parents resisted talking about how they felt about a Do Not Resuscitate (DNR) order, so one day he mentioned to them that a person of very advanced age had gone in for knee surgery and died of an infection while in the hospital. His father's response was, "I can't believe he went in for that surgery at his age. Hadn't he ever heard of 'death by hospital?'"

That told his son all he needed to hear. His father was definitely in favor of a DNR, and that comment led to an extended conversation about setting up the order for him. I recommend this indirect method of broaching delicate topics if your loved ones resist talking about them. Talk to them about other people and the decisions they've made regarding Do Not Resuscitate orders in living wills, and then ask your loved one for their opinion or preferences.

My experience is that most older adults want to do the things that make them happy later in life, whether it's reading novels, having a bowl of ice cream every night, taking walks, or sipping wine while watching movies.

If they can't do the things that make them happy and are faced with being confined to bed or a wheelchair, they may not want to prolong their lives under those conditions.

Knowing how your parents feel about having a DNR order in place is particularly important. If they have a serious medical problem at any point, one of the first things you will be asked by the EMTs or the ER nurse is, "Do they have a DNR?"

This is not a cut and dry matter. It is a quiet secret in the emergency medical field that older people often do not survive an attempt at resuscitation. And, if they do, they often sustain serious injuries. We've all watched television shows where the EMT tries to get a patient's heart beating regularly again either with manual CPR or with a defibrillator. Older people often suffer crushed ribs and other injuries during those resuscitation techniques, so even if their heartbeats are restored, their health will be seriously compromised.

Many people also think that if they have a living will, they're all set. But that only works if two physicians agree that you have a terminal diagnosis. So, for example, if your parent, who is fragile and has memory impairment, slips and falls and incurs bleeding in the brain, the ER docs and surgeons will likely want to go in and do a procedure to stop the bleeding. Because your parent didn't have a terminal diagnosis, all efforts were taken to prolong their life.

But that is a major surgery requiring anesthesia, which can make memory impairment even more severe and seriously impact quality of life. The doctors will argue that if they don't repair the bleed, the patient might have a stroke. But no one really knows what will happen with the operation, because they don't do medical studies on people in their eighties. The saying is that those in that age group are "evidence free" because clinical trials and studies are only done on much younger people.

In my forty years of working with older people, I've never had someone say, "I want to spend my final years incapacitated in a nursing home."

The tough decisions come when there is no terminal diagnosis, but you have to decide on medical intervention. With patients in their eighties, there is a 90 percent chance that surgery will result in a decline in condition and quality of life.

The health care system, which is focused on fixing, curing, and treating for a profit, will push you to "treat for a cure." But they make money doing procedures, and most of the time, they will not answer the question: "What would you do if this was your parent?" Or other questions such as these:

"Will the person still be able to walk? Go to the bathroom alone? Eat alone?"

Locate, Organize, and Update Personal Paperwork

Marty and Nancy were in their late eighties. He was living at home, but Nancy had moved into a nearby assisted living facility with some health issues. Then, at the height of the Covid-19 pandemic, Marty was stopped by a police officer while driving. He appeared confused and was found to have an impaired memory.

Their daughter, who lived out of the area, called our company to assess the situation and make recommendations for the couple's care. We found that Marty did not want to move into an assisted living home, but clearly, he needed to. So, we moved him into the same place as his wife because it had a special unit for those with memory impairment.

Marty was not a happy camper there. His primary pastime was escaping and trying to return to their former home. His actions made it clear that Marty was no longer capable of managing the couple's financial and legal affairs, nor was he able to make good decisions regarding their health care.

Now, Nancy had power of attorney for her husband, but most of the time, you cannot take that role over unless you have a document from a medical professional establishing that your spouse no longer has the mental capacity to act on his own behalf.

My team had to run all over the place during the coronavirus pandemic to get letters and legal documents signed and certified. This involved trying to find, assemble, and organize the couple's financial, legal, and medical records, which was no simple task.

Prepare to Become an Advocate

There have been even more complications in this case involving Nancy's deteriorating physical and mental condition, but the point here is that handling this series of crises would have been much easier for all parties if the couple's paperwork had been assembled and organized for easy access.

Critical decisions about securing power of attorney and hiring health care surrogates requires legal and medical documentation. Family members should have contact information for their parent's lawyers—especially those who have their wills on file—and their primary doctor. The doctors and attorneys should have you registered in their files as someone approved by the parents to receive otherwise confidential medical and legal information.

The same holds true with your parent's bank and financial advisors. They have their own processes for approving your power of attorney so that you can write checks out of their accounts or withdraw money to pay for their expenses. You'll also want to have access to any stocks, mutual funds, IRAs, or other financial instruments. Some will ask for documentation from your parent's doctors saying that the individual no longer has the mental capacity to handle their own affairs.

If this seems like a lot to handle, it is, and you really don't want to be trying to set all of this up at the last minute. Believe me, I've been called in to handle these matters for clients during times of family crisis. There is no hurrying banks, lawyers, and physician's staff just because you need documentation as soon as possible.

While it might be a difficult conversation to have when your parent is still independent and doing well, you will be very glad to have prepared for the fragile years ahead and all the challenges they bring. Find out if your parents have a living will stating preferences on life-prolonging medical procedures, funeral services, internment, and distribution of their remaining assets and belongings upon passing. If they do not have a living will and haven't documented their preferences for funeral services, internment, and asset distribution, you should encourage them to do that.

It's certainly not anything most people want to do, but the alternative is to have someone else determine it for you after you are gone, and no one is ever happy with the way that goes.

You should also determine if they have someone in mind among family members or friends to serve as their power of attorney if that becomes necessary.

Have your loved one help you gather critical information on wills, preferred funeral and burial arrangements, bank and investment accounts, health and life insurance, medical records, loan and mortgage accounts.

Other important paperwork includes property titles and deeds, car titles, online passwords and pin numbers, loan papers, investment information, and monthly bills for household expenses and insurance. Find out where they have stored important records including information on health and life insurance, bank and investment accounts, medical records, and mortgage and other outstanding loans.

Your Takeaway Tips:

- *Begin preparing yourself and your parent for the fragile years as they enter their seventies.*
- *Gather critical information on wills, preferred funeral and burial arrangements, bank and investment accounts, health and life insurance, medical records, loan and mortgage accounts.*
- *While your parent is still mentally fit, discuss their preferences for the late stages of life, especially their feelings and preferences regarding life-sustaining procedures and where they prefer to spend their final days. Use examples of other people and what they did if loved ones won't open up about themselves.*

- *As your parent approaches the fragile years, contact several local nursing homes and get to know the staff members on a personal level. Be aware that there is a chronic shortage of beds in nursing homes. Find out how many long-term beds are available. Cultivate contacts at each local facility so they will notify you when beds may be available. Keep it personal!*
- *If your parent is resistant to any help, search for a trusted advisor: care managers are trained to provide help in these types of scenarios. It is money well spent.*
- *Find out where your parent keeps important documents and secure them all in a place or places where you can get to them. These include property titles and deeds, car titles, online passwords and pin numbers, loan papers, investment information, and monthly bills for household expenses and insurance.*
- *Do not buy into the "role reversal" concept that says you have become the parent, and your parent has become the child. That attitude will only result in bitterness and resentment. Remain respectful and patient, treat your parent the way you will want your children to treat you as you age. There is no role reversal; that is a recipe for making your parents angry at you.*
- *Make the most of the time you have remaining with your loved one. This is your opportunity to create even more meaningful memories and to let them know once again that they are loved and will be remembered.*

Chapter Four

Finding a Caring Place for Your Parent

After enjoying eighty-five years of good health and independent living, Catherine had a life-changing medical event. The timing of these events is never good, but for Catherine it was especially bad. She was in a hotel room in a city nearly three hundred miles from her home and the small Midwestern town where she'd spent her entire life.

To make matters even worse, Catherine's medical emergency happened on the morning of her granddaughter's wedding, with hundreds of family members and friends gathered to celebrate. She called her daughter from her hotel room and said she felt weak, light-headed, and she was having trouble breathing.

"It feels like my heart is racing, and for some reason, my feet are so swollen I can't get my shoes on," she said.

Her daughter, the mother of the bride, was a veteran nurse, and she recognized the symptoms as being heart-related. She called 911 and had the EMTs take her mother to a local hospital. The ER doctors diagnosed a faulty heart valve.

The hospital's cardiologist urged her to have the heart valve repaired in a surgery. Catherine, who was widowed, had been playing golf, volunteering at church and community events, and enjoying an active social life up to that point.

She believed the cardiologists when they told her that she could return to that independent and active lifestyle after the surgery. Still sharp-minded and alert, Catherine was capable of making her own decision.

Her nurse daughter cautioned her that recovery might be difficult for a woman of her years. Yet Catherine noted that her own mother had lived to be 103, so she had no reason to believe that wouldn't be true for her.

"I still have a lot of time left and I want to enjoy it," she said.

The hospital had a good reputation. It was an urban medical center, a teaching hospital, that was much more well-equipped and well-staffed than the small hospital in her rural hometown. So, she decided to have the surgery to repair her faulty heart valve there.

I will write in more depth in a later chapter about the high risks involved with surgery for patients in their eighties and above, but sad to say, Catherine would prove to be one of those who was never able to recover the life she'd had after her operation.

Yet, her case is all too common. After her surgery, which was successful in repairing the heart valve, Catherine experienced a series of other health problems. As a result of the operation, she was put on a ventilator, and there was scarring on her throat.

Attempts to remove the ventilator and repair the damage were unsuccessful. She never again was independent of the ventilator. When the hospital wanted to discharge her, Catherine's children scrambled to find her a caring place that would take her on a ventilator.

They quickly realized that the vast majority of nursing homes would not take someone on a ventilator. Nor would any assisted living centers. They did find one nursing home willing to accept her, but it was hundreds of miles from family and friends in a very remote corner of the state.

To their great fortune, one of Catherine's children knew a family of doctors and surgeons closer to home who owned and operated a rural hospital with attached nursing home and assisted living facilities. These kind friends made an exception to their usual rules and accepted Catherine.

"I will take care of her as if she were my own mother," their doctor friend told them. And he lived up to that promise. His attentive staff kept Catherine in an intensive care unit where they cared for her for five months until she passed peacefully, surrounded by family.

The Challenges of Finding a Caring Place

Most families are not so fortunate, sadly. Unless they have a plan in place before a crisis occurs, most have to settle for whatever bed they can find. Adult children with aging parents often have the misguided belief that, when the time comes, they will easily find their loved one a lovely nursing home just down the street with a great rehab center and caring staff.

That is rarely possible. In many areas, there simply are not enough nursing home beds to meet growing demand. This was especially true during the Covid-19 epidemic, and it is a continuing issue with the aging of the Baby Boomer generation. Most facilities have two patients in a room, and the majority of residents are women, so finding a fragile older male a nursing home bed is especially challenging.

If a parent can't live independently in their own homes any longer, most people want to find residential care somewhere near their home and family. So, location is a consideration, but cost is an even greater factor for most people. Quality of care is another critical consideration.

If the individual has or develops mental or memory impairment due to Alzheimer's or other forms of dementia, the challenges can be even greater—particularly if their behavior is challenging (wandering or aggression) and the need is for nursing home care. The nursing home is highly regulated, and there are not many nursing homes specializing in memory care with dedicated memory units.

Assisted living is different because there are many with memory units these days. Even so, their higher costs can put these units out of reach for many families. My advice is always to keep that in mind when looking at any facility, particularly if there is a family history of memory impairment.

I will write more about those specific challenges later, but one thing to keep in mind is that if your parent has even mild or early-stage dementia, you may have to move them to another place if it progresses, unless their current facility has a memory care unit to accommodate them. This is especially true in continuing care retirement communities.

Activities of Daily Living

It's important to know some basic definitions when entering the world of assisted living centers and nursing homes and the levels of care each provides.

Instrumental Activities of Daily Living (IADLs) are the tasks that can be done by someone living independently. They include using the telephone, driving, shopping, taking medication, and housekeeping.

Activities of Daily Living (ADLs) are basic self-care activities such as bathing, grooming, dressing, toileting, eating, and transferring/mobility.

The other concept to grasp is that of assistance and dependence. When an older person needs assistance with bathing or dressing but is otherwise capable of most tasks, the first option would be assisted living. If the individual becomes unable to use the bathroom or perform other self-care, then the next move would be into a nursing home, in most cases.

Making the distinction as to the level of care required can be very subjective and hard to define; many children think that their parent is dependent when they just need assistance and vice versa. Additionally, in some states, assisted living communities can provide care that is dependent care under a special additional license.

Let's look at the various types of long-term residential care facilities and what they offer.

Assisted Living

Residents of assisted living centers, also known in some states as personal care homes, typically need more hands-on help with daily life, though not as much as is provided in a nursing home. There are small (five bed) communities and larger communities with over one hundred units. They can be homes in residential communities or large apartment style communities with different sizes of apartments.

When an older person needs assistance with one or more daily activities such as bathing, dressing, using the toilet, eating, walking, and transferring from bed to a chair, (or wheelchair or walker) to bed and back, then that individual meets the requirement for admission into an assisted living center.

Some communities offer all-inclusive pricing, but most charge a base rate which covers room and board, meals, activities, limited transportation, housekeeping, maintenance, and minimal assistance with care.

Levels of care (three or four levels at $200–$300 per level) are offered depending on the care needs of the resident. There are various ways to calculate care needs. Some use a point system. Others might have fees for specific kinds of care such as assisting those who are incontinent or have memory issues. Special needs like those increase the level of care required and the cost of providing it.

It's important to understand how the community you are considering calculates the level of care so you can be sure it's affordable for your family member. The monthly costs can range widely depending on the level of care provided, the size and credentials of the staff, and the state where the center is located. Shared rooms are available at a lower cost. Typically, smaller homes are less expensive than larger communities. The least expensive might be $3,000 to $4,000 a month in Florida for assisted living care, with the fees increasing to more than $6,000 a month for memory care.

Assisted living care costs are higher in the northeast and Alaska, with the US average at $4,000. In the larger communities, residents have their own apartments with access to common areas. Services provided usually include three meals daily, personal care, housekeeping and laundry, twenty-four-hour staff and security on site. Social and recreational programs are usually offered.

If your parent wants to bathe every day rather than twice a week, which is standard, you should arrange for that with the staff and see what the additional cost is. Often, a resident will become more in need of assistance while in an assisted living facility, which requires a move to a nursing home eventually.

Some assisted living centers do not provide help with certain tasks like assisting residents with putting on medically-prescribed support-hose, which requires training. So, you might have to pay extra to have someone come in and help them with those tasks.

Residents with arthritic hands may have trouble zipping up pants or buttoning blouses and shirts, or putting on belts, which may move them to a higher level of care. Those seem like such standard daily tasks, but imagine how much time it would take if staff members had to do those things for every resident.

If your loved one can no longer perform those basic tasks at all or help with any part of it, then the person may need to move to a nursing home. Assisted living centers are not well-regulated, so there is little uniformity in facilities across the nation.

Regulations and requirements vary from state to state in assisted living communities because there are no federal laws governing them. This lack of federal oversight has become an issue as more and more of these facilities are built nationwide. The building boom is due to the fact that assisted living facilities are more profitable than nursing homes for the owners.

That is why big corporations are getting into the assisted living center business. One phenomenon I have noticed is that when they first open, many assisted living centers have great staffing and programs, but after a while, they may reduce staffing and programs to cut costs. Or they might swap out a higher salary registered nurse for a licensed practical nurse. The lower the level of medical care, the more vigilant family members will need to be in monitoring their loved ones who live there.

One thing to look for: most assisted living centers provide call bells for residents to summon staff from their beds. These are provided mostly for emergency situations. If your loved one is ringing the call bell several times a day for help with non-emergency things like getting dressed or using the restroom, then it might be time to move them to a nursing home that provides a higher level of care.

Family members and residents are often shocked to learn that most assisted living facilities are based on "social" models, meaning the emphasis is on the living environment, rather than medical models of care. That is a good thing to keep in mind.

If your loved one has one or more medical issues, you should make certain that there is a registered nurse (RN) or a licensed vocational nurse (LVN) on the property seven days a week to manage their care. Not many of these facilities meet that requirement. If there is a nurse on staff, you might also inquire as to how many residents that nurse is responsible for at any given time.

So, when you are looking at assisted living centers for your loved one, or for yourself, take the time to check what level of care they provide. You might also ask for references from residents or the family members of residents.

Key Questions to Ask About Assisted Living Centers:

* What level of nursing care do they provide? Do they have a registered nurse or a licensed practical nurse on duty, and how many hours per day and how many days per week?

- How many residents is the nurse responsible for during each shift?
- How many aides are on staff? What are their certification requirements?
- What is the aide-to-resident ratio for each shift?
- Ask to talk to a new resident and someone who has been there for a while.
- Solicit feedback from families who are visiting.
- Read the survey reports (most states will survey quality of care).
- How long has the current administrator been working there, and how many administrators have been employed over the last ten years?
- Who administers medications to patients, and what is their training? Many of these facilities now assign that job not to nurses but to "med techs" who have only six to eight hours of training. If a resident is taking more than a few medications, this can be problematic because the med techs are only trained to pass out pills. They don't have training in how combining certain meds can impact a resident's health.

In addition, a med tech does not have the skills that a nurse would have to evaluate a person's drug regimen and medical history when discussing that individual with a primary physician.

Assisted Living Centers Do Not Keep Medical Records of Residents

Be aware also that assisted living centers are not required to keep medical records and charts like hospitals and nursing homes. Adult children are sometimes surprised to check in on their parents and find there are no medical records available. They simply don't keep them and in many states aren't required to.

If your parent is sent to the hospital from an assisted living center, the center does not always send along medical information for the admissions staff to review. Sometimes, they might send the medication list. So, it is important for you to have up to date information on your parents to provide to the hospital. Also, the facility does not send staff members to the hospital with residents.

This is especially fraught for those with memory impairment, so it is even more challenging to navigate. It helps to have someone advocating for your loved one.

That is why I advise family members to have at least a brief overview of a loved one's list of meds, allergies, and other vital medical information in case they get sent to an ER from an assisted living center that can't easily and quickly provide that information.

In some states there are regulations that do not allow assisted living facilities to provide services like an insulin injection or managing their oxygen. You might have to pay an aide or someone else to come in and provide those services if your loved one needs them.

The pattern over the years is that older people are waiting longer to move into assisted living centers, which means the residents often are more frail and in poorer health than in the past. So, the quality of medical care available and the number of staff available to assist residents has become more important.

More and more assisted living centers have several levels of care so that you can move up to a higher level—at a higher price—without leaving the facility. I had one client with both parents in an assisted living home. His mother was on a lower level of care than his father. The cost was an additional $400 a month for the father's care.

However, my client noticed that her mother was doing most of those "extra" things that were supposed to be provided by staff, including feeding and bathing her husband. So, the client had me renegotiate the amount she'd been paying for the father's care.

My advice is to always monitor the level of care your loved one is receiving, to make sure the facility is providing what you are paying for. It can be very subjective, and needs can change.

If your parent goes into the hospital for surgery and comes back to the assisted living home needing rehabilitation services, then that will require a higher level and probably cost more, but then, once the parent has recuperated, the level of care should go down and the cost, too.

Nursing Homes

Most people are familiar with the term "nursing home" and what it means. Nursing homes are also referred to as "skilled nursing facilities," "rehab facilities," or "health and rehabilitation centers."

I'll stick with "nursing home" just to keep it simple. Medicare covers rehabilitation (physical, occupational, speech, and respiratory therapy) which is provided in skilled nursing facilities. The modern version typically includes "rehab" wings for short-term stays and long-term care wings for permanent residents.

Rehab wings are for those older people who are recovering from health problems or medical procedures. They stay in this wing to receive services from licensed professionals only long enough to recover, so they can then return to their former residence.

You may hear references to short-term beds or long-term beds, and that is what they are referring to. The long-term care residents are there for the remainder of their lives because it is the most affordable place to live given the high level of care they require.

Nursing homes offer a greater range and depth of care and services than assisted living centers. The nursing home provides dependent care when a person is totally dependent on someone to accomplish one or more of their ADLs. For that reason, they are required to have nurses on staff twenty-four hours per day.

Physical, occupational, and speech therapists are also provided for short-term residents, and under Medicare criteria, some long-term residents can receive therapy as well.

Unlike assisted living centers, nursing homes are heavily regulated. Nursing home administrators like to say that their facilities are the second most regulated of all industries, while noting that the first is the nuclear power industry.

I have seen the industry become more regulated over the years, requiring a lot of management staff because of all the rules, but the aide to patient ratio has stayed basically the same. If we could change that around and require a higher aide to patient ratio, the care in nursing homes would be so much better.

For the aging people looking for a caring place to live in their fragile years—and the loved ones assisting them—the challenges of navigating the system are complicated by the fact that this is not only heavily regulated but deeply fragmented.

As I noted earlier, those fragments, or "silos" include hospitals and pharmacies, nursing homes, including short-term and long-term care, assisted living centers, home-care, hospices, and the often-baffling web of the health insurance industry, including Medicare, Medicaid, and veterans' benefits.

I will write more in later chapters about the challenges of moving between and among those silos when a loved one enters the fragile years. For now, let me offer you some insights on nursing homes and what they offer.

Rehabilitation Hospitals or Inpatient Rehabilitation

If an older patient has been hospitalized and is ready for discharge, the hospital staff social worker, nurse, or physician might recommend that the patient be sent to a rehabilitation hospital. Rehabilitation hospitals are specialty hospitals, or a part of larger acute care hospitals, that offer intensive inpatient rehabilitation therapy.

Your loved one may need inpatient care in a rehabilitation hospital if recovering from a serious illness, surgery, or injury. This level of care cannot be provided in the home or a skilled nursing facility.

Examples of common conditions that may qualify someone for care in a rehabilitation hospital include stroke, spinal cord injury, and brain injury. They may not qualify for care if, as an example, recovering from hip or knee replacement with no other complicating condition.

Rehab hospitals provide aggressive therapy (four to six hours daily) and can produce remarkable results. This may not be the best option for an elder in their fragile years because they cannot tolerate the amount of therapy given, they might not want to work that hard, and the discharge plan from the hospital must be to their home, not to a nursing home.

Choosing a Nursing Home

My first piece of advice when choosing a nursing home is to find out what the inventory of long-term beds is in your community. How many nursing homes are in the area? How many have long-term beds available?

This is the most important piece of information and will affect all decisions you make. It is dizzying to try and figure out this information, so again, I would recommend hiring a care manager who will be able to help you understand and guide you through the nursing home search so you can find the best possible place for your loved one.

Other Critical Factors to Consider:

- Location: If you have a choice of nursing homes, I like to have my clients live near family if possible. This allows frequent visits to check on the needs and wants of your parent.
- Affordability: Are the costs of the nursing home affordable for the individual? Do they accept Medicaid when the family funds run out?
- Access to the outdoors

- Do they have private rooms on campus, and can you get on the waiting list?
- How long have the administrator and the director of nursing worked there?
- It is important to try and match the primary needs of your parent with what the facility does well. For example, if your parent is extroverted and socially active, how are the activities programs? How long has the activity director worked there, and how well attended are their programs?
- If the quality of the meals is important to the loved one, I suggest having a meal there before signing up to see how good it is—or not.

Keep in mind what sort of activities they enjoy and whether they are introverted or extroverted. Some care facilities are more aggressive than others in encouraging residents to participate in programs and activities.

I learned also that an older person can surprise you, even in their fragile years. I never would have imagined that my father would become an avid bingo player, but darned if he didn't sign up and go to every session he could.

Bingo may get a bad rap, but it's actually a good brain exercise to keep several cards going at once while listening to the bingo caller and staying stimulated by your fellow players.

Remember that your loved one may need time to adjust to the new living environment. Some may balk at activities at first, but eventually enjoy them. I had an "introverted" client who spent her days watering plants, folding laundry, feeding other residents, and becoming the unofficial mayor of the nursing home.

Many older people find that once they settle into a nursing home, they feel more secure and calmer, especially if they are having memory issues or a fear of falling at home alone. They may not have noticed how anxious they were about living alone until that burden is eased.

Others become depressed, feeling like life is not worth living, and lose interest in everything.

Checklist for Nursing Homes

Things to look for when checking out nursing homes include:

- The staff to resident ratio on each shift: how many aides on 7-3, 3-11, and 11-7
- The size of the budget
- Its reputation among residents, their families, and the local community
- What is the staff turnover per category (nurses, aides, housekeeping, maintenance, and management)
- Visit at different times of the day and different days of the week. What is the facility like on the weekend?
- Note how the staff interacts with residents. Do they know their names? Have conversations with them? Seem attentive to their needs?
- Do the residents seem to be content, or are they anxious? Do they interact with each other or seem isolated?
- Are the residents out of bed mid-morning?
- Can your loved one stay with you over a weekend?
- Do physicians work in the facility? How many patients are assigned to them? How many facilities do they work with?

Do they work with advanced registered nurse practitioners or physician's assistants?

- Is a transportation service available for doctor or hospital visits?
- Is there a van to take residents to appointments or shopping?
- Are the resident's rooms suited to your parent's needs and desires?
- Are they allowed to bring in their favorite pieces of furniture? Are televisions furnished?
- What accommodations are made for those who are hard of hearing or vision impaired?
- Do the rooms have pleasant views?
- Do the residents seem happy, clean, appropriately dressed and well-groomed at a decent time of day?
- What specialty medical services are provided? This is important if your parent is on dialysis or has a tracheotomy. If your parent is on a ventilator, it will become extremely difficult no matter where you live to find a nursing home.
- Nursing homes are surveyed annually. The report should be easily found in the facility or online. Read it to see what the problem areas have been.
- Are safety measures like handrails, smoke detectors, sprinklers, and grab bars in bathrooms in good working order?
- Can residents choose from a menu or custom-order meals? Can they eat alone in their rooms if they wish?
- Does the kitchen seem clean and well-organized? Do they offer a wide range of meals? Are snacks and drinks available to residents at all times? What activities are offered? Is

there outdoor space for recreation? Does the facility offer excursions or outings for residents?

Your loved one might have friends or family in nearby care facilities, or they might have heard of others recommended by friends. Check them out. Ask for references from residents and their families. Contact several local nursing homes and get to know the staff members on a personal level.

As I mentioned earlier, there is a chronic shortage of beds in nursing homes. So make sure you find out how many long-term beds are available. Cultivate contacts at each local facility so they will notify you when beds may be available. Keep it personal!

The Cost of Nursing Home Care

Nursing homes cost more than assisted living centers because of the greater range and depth of care they provide. If you can find a private room, it can cost (according to Genworth, a company specializing in long-term care insurance) from $8,346 a month, or $275 per day. A semi-private room starts at $7,441 a month, or $244 per day.

There is a large difference in nursing home costs across the country. Length of stay, extra services you might need, and available amenities can also impact the cost. Those individuals requiring memory care units will require more expensive care.

Those cost figures can seem daunting, but there are ways to reduce some of your expenses with tax deductions, life and long-term care insurance, VA benefits, and Medicaid.

I've discovered that some clients have life insurance policies that can be sold on a secondary market, which can help fund nursing home care. That is an important thing to check on!

My favorite example of this is a client we worked with who had thirty-seven life insurance policies! Yes, it was a record that still stands in our company. We could not believe it. The point is that if your parents have life insurance policies with death benefits of, say, $200,000, you can sell those on a secondary market, and that cash might open up new options for them.

Your life insurance is considered an asset that can be sold. You can get an expert broker to examine it and put a value on it, then you can offer it to buyers who specialize in this market.

Selling your life insurance is like selling any other asset you own. You ask a third party to look at the policy and value it, then take your policy to a group of buyers, and someone will offer to buy it from you. Typically, the buyers are big banks and financial institutions such as JP Morgan, Deutsche Bank, or AIG.

Keep in mind that the insurance companies that sell those policies just love it when people file for Medicaid because then they have to get rid of their life insurance policies. We work with a company called WorthRight to help our clients value and sell their life insurance policies if that is an option they want to pursue. It's sad that so few people realize this is an option because thousands don't realize the value of them, and they simply surrender their life insurance policies instead of using that money to pay for care.

Another issue we run into is that many times family members assume that Medicare will pay for nursing home care, but you can only get Medicaid if you have "spent down" all of your money, and if you weren't a career military person, you can't get VA benefits.

Medicare only covers certain specific skilled care expenses related to medical and rehab treatment while you are in a nursing home and the room and board charges associated with that short-term stay. For example, if a long-term resident returns from a surgery or other medical procedure in a hospital or clinic, Medicare will pay for short-term care, but only if the person was:

* In the hospital for at least three days. (Because of Covid care requirements, this criterion has been lifted temporarily.)
* Admitted into a Medicare certified facility within thirty days of the hospitalization.
* Needs physical or speech therapy or other forms of rehab.

Under those very specific conditions, Medicare covers up to twenty days of care in a skilled nursing facility, and then will cover 80 percent of the bill, leaving a co-pay of $176 per day up to the 100th day after admission. After that 100-day mark, all Medicare coverage ends, so the individual must pay out of pocket.

After eligibility is secured, Medicaid will pay 100 percent (less a person's income) of the costs of care in a nursing home. Military veterans with injuries or disabilities incurred during their service usually have full coverage as part of their Veterans Affairs benefits within a veteran's skilled nursing facility or any other skilled nursing facility that has a contract with the Veteran's Administration. Even those vets who do not have disabilities related to their military service can qualify for VA benefits, which we will discuss in Chapter Nine.

Important Tips for Navigating the Maze

Your monthly fees for room and board and medical care in a nursing home are tax deductible if you are living there primarily for medical care, which presumably you are. The material above is the basic nuts and bolts information on Medicare, Medicaid, and VA benefits for nursing home residents. Now, I want to give you some additional tips that you may find helpful, based on my many years of dealing with this complex and often frustrating system.

Those with less than $2,000 in assets and under $2,349 in 2020 in monthly income can qualify for the Medicaid Institutional Care Program (ICP) to pay nursing home costs.

Although there is an income limit for ICP Medicaid, there are ways (legal!) around the income limit for this program in certain states that allow "qualified income trusts." A qualified income trust is an income-only trust, drafted by an attorney.

This requires hiring a lawyer to draft a legal document that outlines the person's income. You can then take that document to a bank and open a qualified income trust account. For every month you want Medicaid eligibility, you have to deposit the amount that puts you over the income limit. Money from that trust account can then be paid to the nursing home. Given that all the person's income goes to the nursing, this is typically less, and often far less than what the nursing home would charge.

If the income limit is $2,349 per month, and you make $2,350, every month you pay the nursing home one dollar out of the account. If you miss a month then you are not eligible for Medicaid for that month.

When you are in a nursing home on Medicaid, you are allowed to subtract from your gross income as much as $130 a month from your income for "personal needs" and pay the remainder to the nursing home for your "patient's responsibility," which is basically your rent. You can also subtract the cost of supplemental insurance and dental care if you have those.

States have varying regulations about how assets like your home and your retirement fund can affect your Medicaid eligibility, so you might want to talk to an accountant or an attorney who specializes in "elder law" and protecting your assets. It can get very complicated, but there are strategies that can reduce the costs of staying in a nursing home.

If there is a spouse still at home, this all gets more complicated, especially because the rules vary state to state. In Florida, spouses at home can have a higher income to support themselves if their incomes fall below Medicaid's minimum monthly maintenance needs allowance.

Let's say Doug and Cindy are an older Florida couple. Doug's Social Security check is $1,500 and Cindy's is $1,000. When Doug goes into a nursing home, he qualifies for Medicaid long-term assistance. Cindy's income is below Medicaid's minimum monthly maintenance needs allowance, so she can hang onto at least $1,155 of Doug's monthly income and put the rest toward his nursing home rent.

If you have a hard time following that, don't feel bad. It's very complicated, and the rules often change. I can't give financial advice to clients, but I often direct them to public accountants and lawyers who can help them figure out what is best for them.

Continuing Care Retirement Communities (CCRCs)

Continuing care retirement communities (CCRCs), also known as life plan communities, offer multiple levels of care on one campus: independent living, assisted living, and nursing home care. They feature a variety of other amenities and services such as a clinic nurse, twenty-four-hour security, and emergency alert systems. This appeals to consumers who want to stay in one community as their care needs change and to older adults with no family or no family living close by.

Older adults "buy in" which comes in the form of an entrance fee (ranging from $100,000 to $500,000). These communities often feature resort-style amenities such as meal plans and active lifestyle programs. The big appeal with CCRCs is that once you pay the entrance fees and monthly charges, you have one very nice place to stay for the rest of your life.

They provide several levels of service including independent housing and apartments, assisted living, and skilled nursing care all on one site. Health care services and recreation programs are also provided.

The "continuing care" refers to the fact that residents can move from one level of service to the next within the complex, depending on their needs at any given time. They can live in their own homes or apartments on the grounds, with or without home care as well, or move to the assisted living or nursing home levels.

Most of the good ones are accredited. They typically have an entrance fee program that is amortized at a rate of 2 percent a month so, up to a certain point, if you leave you can get a refund. If you have long-term care insurance, living here might not make sense unless you don't mind being doubly insured.

There is a price for peace of mind. The entry fees range from the low- to mid-six figures or more. Monthly charges are also quite high, from $2,000 to more than $4,000 depending on various factors including whether you live in one of the homes on the grounds or in a one- or two-bedroom apartment. Those costs tend to vary a lot depending on location and amenities and what options and plans you choose.

For example, you can sign a guaranteed refund option contract and pay a higher entry fee that refunds just the entry fee upon death. It covers the costs of care as needed, which protects you and your family financially if you later need to move into assisted living or nursing care. Entrance fees do not cover the cost of care. They offer the security of knowing you will stay within the same community as your care needs change.

It would be important to ask for all contract options offered by a community, including rental agreements. Some continuing care retirement communities offer rental contracts on a limited basis. These don't require an entry fee, but the monthly maintenance fees are higher.

Most CCRCs are set up so that a declining percentage of the entry fee is refunded if an individual leaves or dies within a few years of moving. Some will guarantee a refund percentage for the individual or family heirs if a higher entry fee is paid.

Many continuing care retirement communities are wonderful, particularly those that are near universities or colleges and have affiliations that allow residents to use their facilities. Sometimes called "University Based Retirement Communities" (UBRCs), these college town CCRCs provide access for residents to attend or audit many university classes and events like concerts and sports, while also allowing them to enjoy campus libraries, recreation and fitness centers, and other campus facilities.

Residents often say they enjoy being around young people and the intellectual environment of a college campus—at least during the day. Some of the most noted UBRCs include Oak Hammock in Gainesville, Florida, which is affiliated with the University of Florida; Kendal at Hanover, affiliated with Dartmouth College in New Hampshire; and Holy Cross Village at Notre Dame, affiliated with Holy Cross and St. Mary's Colleges in Indiana.

Expert Advice May Be Required

I would strongly recommend consulting with a financial advisor, a care manager, and an attorney if considering moving into a CCRC. Each profession will give you objective feedback with regard to your finances, the care costs, and understanding the contracts.

You should have a professional review all the available contracts to determine which one fits your financial goals. The older you are, the less it makes sense to pay an entrance fee, as you don't live long enough to take advantage of the discounts for health services in the future. If you have purchased long-term care insurance and want to keep the insurance, it makes even less sense. You may want to cash out your long-term care insurance when moving into a CCRC.

Another consideration: If you have a family history of Alzheimer's or dementia, does the CCRC you are considering have memory care in assisted living and the nursing home? Some do, many do not. It's true that as we get older our cognition is slower and diminished.

Alzheimer's and other forms of dementia can be accompanied by problem behaviors that require extra support in a specialized memory unit. If the CCRC doesn't provide this kind of care and you develop a problematic memory problem, you may be asked to move out.

The first time this happened to a client of mine, her father pulled the fire alarm in the stairwell at 2:00 in the morning. The administrator told my client's daughter that if this behavior continued, he would have to leave the community. A few weeks later he missed his twenty-four-hour security check, and no one knew where he was. He was missing for hours and finally returned unable to tell anyone where he had gone.

The administrator stated that they were unable to care for him safely, and we helped him move into an assisted living community with memory care. He had paid an entrance fee and was ineligible for a refund, and they couldn't care for him because of the lack of memory care on campus.

I had another client living independently in a CCRC who was found in the lobby at 3:00 a.m. wanting to go outside. The security guard called us, and we hired caregivers to stay with her twenty-four hours per day. She continued to wander because she experienced a reversal of day and night. The administrator asked us to move her to the assisted living area so she could be more closely monitored.

Her expressed wish over the years was to never leave her apartment. She could afford twenty-four-hour care. Since the assisted living center did not have a memory support unit, she would have had the same issues there as she did in her apartment.

Given the situation, we supported her decision to stay in her apartment. She had caregivers helping her for the rest of her life.

Additional guidance for those looking at CCRC facilities:

- Tour the assisted living facilities and nursing homes several times on different days and times of day. Ask residents about the quality of care. Check the state's ratings for each of them.

- Remember you are buying into the entire community and need to see the quality of care and lifestyle is the same throughout the community, not just in independent living.

- In most contracts the facility maintains the right to move you to another level of care, even if you don't want to or think you need to.

- The rates increase annually. Check to see what the past increases have been, so you are prepared for the yearly financial increase.

- I'd also recommend that you ask whether there have been monthly fee increases of more than 3 percent in recent years. This will help you understand what your future costs might be. If they are not open to sharing this information, take that into consideration as well.

- Spend a night or two on the grounds to get a feel for what the lifestyle will be like, as well as the quality of the dining room meals and other amenities.

Making the Move to a Caring Place

Moving into residential care can be a difficult and emotional decision, especially for those who feel like they are giving up their independence and active lifestyles.

I've often had clients and their family members fret about moving from large homes into the much smaller apartments in residential care facilities. That is understandable, but I advise them that if the aging person is in the fragile years, the person may come to appreciate a smaller space to care for and navigate.

I believe that a lot of the assisted living communities market to the adult children, and that older adults as a general rule care less about their physical surroundings than their children do.

They will likely find it easier to navigate in a smaller room. There are also common areas where they can go if they want to have more space. I've had many clients start with two bedrooms and move down to a one bedroom or even a studio because they found it easier to live in cozier quarters as they've aged.

Sad feelings and grieving are part of the process when moving from your longtime home into any residential care facility. Most see it as the end of a more active and social life surrounded by friends and family, but it doesn't have to be that way. You can be as active and social as you want to be in residential care, but you also have the option to just enjoy the peace and quiet of a less hectic lifestyle.

The adult children of my clients often feel guilty and sad, too, but this is often the best option for those who are nearing or already in the fragile years when they will become less independent and more at risk.

It is not unusual for an aging parent to spend a few weeks or months in a residential care home and then want to return home or return to independent living. Many are grieving their former lives, which is quite normal, but their adult children and loved ones often freak out and think they have to move them home.

I explain that this is all understandable for those who are approaching or in the fragile years. They feel vulnerable emotionally and physically. They miss their well-established routines of living at home in familiar surroundings. Maybe they miss their card club friends or their church groups because they can't drive to them anymore.

Often they grow impatient and even angry at all of the adjustments that they have to make as they become more dependent on others for their daily care. My father was well into his fragile years and unable to do many things for himself when he called me one day from his nursing home apartment.

"You will never believe what happened to me today," he said. "This gigantic woman came into my room and said I'm giving you a bath! She wouldn't take no for an answer and she scrubbed me really hard!"

My father needed to talk to someone about this experience, and I was glad he called, though I think he was exaggerating both the size of the woman and the harshness of his treatment. Even so, it was jarring to him, and I saw it as a good sign that he was still sharp-minded enough to call me and express his shock.

Family members often think they have to solve every problem for their older relatives when they are in a care facility, but often the best thing we can do is simply listen and encourage them to enjoy the amenities and security provided by the staff.

One of the best things the "support team" of a person in the fragile zone can do is build relationships with the caregivers and other staff so that you can communicate with them easily and stay informed on your loved one's condition. It never hurts to let those caring for your family member know that someone is keeping an eye on them.

Your Takeaway Tips:

- *Most nursing homes do not work with Medicare Advantage (HMO) plans because they can be labor intensive and generally provide lower than traditional Medicare.*

- *Do not pay an entrance fee to a Continuing Care Retirement Community if your parent is over eighty-five. Odds are that you will never get your money's worth.*

- *Nursing homes often say there is a waiting list for admissions, however, most of those on the waiting list have selected another facility or have passed away by the time their name is called up. So do not hesitate to get on their waiting list as it probably is not as long as they are indicating.*

- *If your parent has a complex medical diagnosis, don't move them into an assisted living facility if there is no registered nurse on staff.*

- *When checking out assisted living facilities, ask for the "nurse to resident ratio" to evaluate how much the staff will manage your parent.*

- *Before moving your parent into an assisted living facility, ask if medications are distributed to residents by a nurse or an aide or med techs. Most aides and med techs have very* limited training. In Florida they have six hours of training for med techs—that's about what you get when training at McDonald's, and these med techs are distributing twenty pills to one person sometimes and can't recognize side effects. If your loved one has a lot of medical issues, you don't want them in a place that lacks a qualified medical team.

- If your parent needs daily medical bandage wraps or uses compression stockings, make sure the facility is allowed to provide this service. Some states prohibit them from doing even something as basic as putting on compression stockings. Ask as many questions as you can to make sure they can take care of your parent's specific needs.

Chapter Five

The Home Care Option

I first met Hazel when one of her friends, who'd been acting as her guardian, asked me to evaluate her mental and physical health. The friend, who had power of attorney for this woman, was concerned that she might need to move out of her longtime residence and into a nursing home.

The friend had already taken the car keys from her because of her erratic driving. Hazel, the friend said, was "a little eccentric."

I visited her and found this dear woman to be in a condition that nurses and aging care professionals refer to as "pleasantly confused." This generally describes someone who has very mild cognitive impairment but is not agitated or combative and can manage most daily tasks with a little guidance. These folks are fun to be around because they are just so darned pleasant.

Hazel was a perfect example of someone in that state. She was generally quite content and happy, though she clearly needed some help if she was to stay at home, which was her stated and longtime desire.

When I visited her house, the place was in need of a serious decluttering and reorganizing. The kitchen was particularly interesting. There were cans and packages everywhere on the shelves and counters, but the refrigerator was the highlight.

All of the nooks and crannies and drawers usually meant for milk, eggs, butter, vegetables, and fruits were packed instead with every variety of Reese's Peanut Butter Cups known to mankind. To be honest, I had no idea that Reese's had so many different types of packaged treats.

Hazel had a chocoholic's wildest dream collection of Reese's Peanut Butter Cups, as well as Reese's Pieces, Reese's Crispy Crunchy Bars, Reese's Clusters, Pretzels, White Cups, White Crème Pink Hearts, Snack Mixes, Eggs, Bells, Trees, Thins, Bars, and my personal holiday favorite: "Reester Bunnies."

Seriously, I gained ten pounds just looking at it.

I cracked up and said to Hazel, "Now, I understand why you only have one tooth!"

She laughed and smiled, flashing that tooth. Just darling, though quite clearly confused. I met with the friend Hazel had chosen to look out for her well-being and recommended that we hire a caregiver so she could remain safely at home.

We didn't make any major changes at first, allowing this sweet woman to grow accustomed to her aide. She kept on eating her Reese's Peanut Butter Cups as we slowly introduced her to other, more healthy foods.

The first time she ate an entire sandwich, her aide called me to joyfully share the news.

"I got Hazel to eat an egg sandwich!"

Apologies to the stockholders of Hershey and Reese's candies, but that was a big day!

Hazel had a well-established routine, and the caregiver worked with it for the most part. In the morning, she liked to go to church, sit in the parking lot for a while, walk around the church to feed the squirrels, and then go to her favorite dollar stores, which were those that sold Reese's candy. Then, she enjoyed having lunch somewhere before going home.

"She once told me that church was where she felt closest to her departed husband," her priest told us.

Just on a whim, one of our more creative aides took Hazel to an art class. She loved it, and before long, she was cranking out beautiful watercolor paintings. My company used one as our Christmas card. Hazel's caretaker friend wept when she saw it.

We managed to keep Hazel in her home for four years with her caregivers, starting out with six hours a day, and over the years it increased to twelve hours per day. Our approach with her was to essentially create an assisted living home environment in her own home. At one point, this client had a serious medical issue and had to be hospitalized. She did a brief stint in rehab after an operation and then we took her back home.

As I write this, this lovely woman is now in hospice, peacefully and pleasantly living out her final days. Most people dream of remaining comfortable in their own homes in the last years of their lives. Sadly, few actually can do that for a variety of reasons, including the financial challenges of paying for home care.

Aging in Place

I have also been working with Dianna and Jorge, who both work full time while supporting Dianna's mother, Rita, a widow, who has been living with them for seventeen years.

For fifteen of those years, Rita has had Alzheimer's. Once she was unable to care for herself, Dianna and Jorge began paying $750 a month for her daycare. Then, after working all day, they'd come home to take care of Rita.

Now, that is true compassion and selflessness. I'm sure it is not easy for them to pay that much money every month out of their humble earnings, or to then come home from their day jobs and act as caregivers. Keeping a fragile older parent at home can seem like the ideal option, especially if there is a family member who can be there to assist them and serve as a companion.

You should know that even those in the fragile years may resist the thought of accepting live-in help or even part-time help. Few older adults will immediately embrace having help at home, regardless of what services are provided.

Often, this resistance is based in fear because the older person thinks it is a sign that the end of life is approaching, and they are no longer in control. A client once told me that she saw accepting a caregiver as "the beginning of the end."

My guidance to loved ones and family members is to expect some resistance at first, and then to empathize with the older person. Realize that it may take more than one conversation for the older adult to accept they need help.

Some may never accept it. If your parent is mentally capable of making thoughtful decisions, you may never get a caregiver into the home—at least not without some serious strategizing—until there is a serious medical problem or other issue.

And, maybe not even then! Many adult children have a tough time with this challenge, and understandably so. It's emotionally wrenching to watch a person you love make decisions that you believe will result in them hurting themselves or being forced to move into a care facility.

I give a speech entitled "When Parents Have the Right to Make Bad Decisions" that is all about dealing with this challenge. My suggestion is that the children give up any thought of "controlling" their aging parents and instead work with them to help them feel more comfortable with assistance.

So, what to do? Small steps are best. You might try first hiring someone part time to help with errands and household tasks that the elderly parent doesn't enjoy doing. Some still enjoy cooking for themselves or even mowing the lawn, but you should also monitor them because that can change quickly for many older people as their energy fades.

I had a ninety-four-year-old client named Ethel with macular degeneration who mowed her lawn every week and prepared her own food. Her son actually bought her a lawn mower for her ninety-fourth birthday. She was delighted and talked about that present with everyone in her church and her circle of friends.

When my team was hired to get her help, we first offered to handle tasks like driving her to church and doing her laundry—two things she couldn't do for herself and did not enjoy. We also got her special reading equipment so she could read the paper every day. Over time, she accepted more and more help from our caregiving team.

Now, there are challenges to this approach—particularly because it is difficult to find skilled home care workers willing to work part-time or just four hours a week. As a general rule, there is more staff turnover for part time work than full time.

If your loved one has a memory impairment, there is almost always resistance to home care workers. My advice is to work around this by saying the care worker is actually a family friend volunteering to help out. This isn't lying. It's diplomacy. And as the decision maker for your loved one, you are responsible for substituting your judgment for their own.

Home Caregivers

If your loved one becomes fragile or has medical problems and you have to hire someone to be with them, hiring a home caregiver is an alternative to moving them into a care facility, however, this can be a more complicated and expensive proposition.

There are different types of home care providers who provide varying levels of service. At the most basic level are personal home care aides, also referred to as non-medical caregivers. They are not highly trained or licensed but can help around the house, run errands, take the client to appointments or shopping, and make meals.

What caregivers can do varies widely from state to state, and the regulations usually revolve around whether someone needs "hands on care," meaning physically bathing and dressing them.

This ongoing service is not covered by Medicare and supplemental insurance. There are times temporary help with a bath is provided while receiving Medicare rehabilitation services, but once the Medicare service ends, the help from the caregiver ends. Payment for caregiver services is a private pay service, and the cost for that ranges widely around the country.

Aides who work for agencies that receive reimbursement from Medicare or Medicaid must get a minimum level of training and pass a competency evaluation to be certified. Some states allow aides to take a competency exam in order to become certified without taking any training.

Additional requirements for certification vary by state. In some states, the only requirement for employment is on-the-job training, which employers generally provide. Other states require formal training, which is available from community colleges, vocational schools, elder care programs, and home health care agencies. In addition, states may conduct background checks on prospective aides. For specific state requirements, contact the state's health board.

Certified Nursing Assistants

You might also consider hiring a certified nursing assistant (CNA), who has more training requirements. A CNA's role typically involves assisting patients with activities of daily living, basic tasks that include bathing, grooming, toileting, eating, and moving. CNAs also fulfill an important role on a patient's health care team since they're often responsible for taking a patient's vital signs.

CNAs offer help with bathing and bathroom routines, and some household tasks like serving meals and changing bedding. They will typically make a dollar or two per hour more than home health care aides.

Nurses

The highest levels of home care providers are either registered nurses (RNs) or licensed practical nurses (LPNs), which also are called licensed vocational nurses (LVNs) in some states. LPNs and LVNs have about a year of training and receive a certificate upon completion of the course and test.

RNs have a license and either a two-year or four-year degree. They have more extensive training in health care and safety and must be licensed by the state. They perform more specialized health care in the home including managing IV tubes, giving injections, tube feeding, diabetic and wound care, and medical assessments. They do not provide domestic services or serve meals in most cases.

At the top of this home care staffing pyramid are registered nurses who have college degrees and have passed national exams and state licensing requirements. They don't do the dishes, but they do provide a high level of medical home care, for which they are well compensated—usually $34.00 an hour or more.

The Costs of Home Care

Caregivers can help ease the loneliness of clients who may not have family or friends nearby. However, the adult children or loved ones of elderly clients often come to us with the misconception that Medicare covers the cost of those aides living or working in shifts in the home. That is not true, unfortunately.

The confusion stems from the fact that Medicare does pay for a specified number of home treatment sessions that are prescribed by a doctor and performed by licensed professionals like registered nurses, or physical, speech, and occupational therapists. Their visits have to be ordered by a physician as part of a treatment program.

In some cases, Medicare will pay for aides to come in three times a week to provide services like baths but only for an hour or so per visit. Medicare does not pay for live-in or day care aides who are there to serve as companions, prepare meals, and do light house-keeping while monitoring the fragile person's health and safety.

Most home health workers who are not nurses provide a range of services including:

- Bathing, dressing, and personal care
- Diet monitoring and meal preparation
- Medication reminders
- Transfer assistance
- Safety checks
- Caregiver relief

You should investigate what the going rates are for home care workers in your area to make sure you aren't over or underpaying them. We also caution clients to be very careful in paying their home care aides. Some might claim to be private or independent contractors and request cash payments so they don't have to pay taxes.

I have observed that clients have varying attitudes on how to hire caregivers. Some have a fear of the IRS "coming after them" if they don't follow IRS rules. Others seem to have no problem with home caregivers who do not pay taxes on their income.

Some clients are very afraid of an accident occurring in their home and want insurance coverage from an outside company to take care of those issues. Others are not so concerned about that.

There are pros and cons with all the options for hiring home caregivers, and I find that giving clients the risks and benefits with each scenario helps individuals decide for themselves which approach feels right for them.

Be aware also that some states require you to buy insurance that covers workers' compensation and disability benefits. You also might want to check with your insurance agent to make sure your homeowner's policy covers the medical and legal costs if your home care aide is injured on the job.

Now, an alternative approach would be to hire a third-party company that can handle all of the back office support needed (recruiting, payroll taxes, IRS reporting, HR requirements).

A third alternative could be to use a professional care manager to recruit candidates, conduct background checks, and make safe referrals to third-party companies or a list of recommendations for you to handle this on your own.

An aging life care agency can manage all of these responsibilities including background screening, hiring and firing, tax and legal documentation. There will likely be added costs, so keep that in mind.

Three Sources for Caregiving Services in the Home

Care management companies like mine provide caregivers who have been properly trained and vetted. You can also find them by asking for referrals from friends and family members, physicians, or local agencies that provide services for the aging. There are also staffing agencies in most cities. You can find them through your local Area Agency on Aging or the listings provided by the National

Association for Home Care & Hospice. Online sources include Care.com and ElderCare.com.

While they charge for their services, these companies provide background checks on home caregivers. Most agencies have a deep pool of experienced caregivers, making it more likely that they can find a good match for your loved one. They also will provide replacements to fill in for your caregiver when needed.

Typically these companies carry insurance that covers the costs if a caregiver is injured in your home. Its administrators handle payment, scheduling, and taxes.

There are also home health care staffing services or registries that help families connect with independent home health care workers based on the needs of your aging at home loved one.

The staff represented by registries are 1099 employees (independent contractors), so there is no insurance coverage. Each staff member handles their own taxes. The company is not allowed to supervise these staff members because they are subcontractors. Most provide background checks and screening and replacement services when there is a staff call out.

Finally, many people find caregivers and hire them privately. They track them down through referrals from friends and family members. Many use care managers to recruit good candidates, or online websites whereby caregivers are listed with their backgrounds and experience. Some of these hires match up well and work for many years with a family.

Keep in mind when caregiving services are provided privately—either through a registry or personal referral—there must be some oversight to prevent exploitation, blurred boundaries, and undue dependency issues causing friction with the family. Every now and then, we hear of cases in which unscrupulous independent home care workers may take advantage of their aging clients and betray the trust put in them.

My company recommends that you always have a trusted family member, friend, or professional monitor their activities and make sure they do not use their positions to manipulate their clients or to steal from them.

I always suggest that at least one trusted family member be put in charge of tracking the aging loved one's credit card accounts as well as checking, savings, and retirement accounts on a regular basis to watch for any indications of unusual transactions.

Your Takeaway Tips:

- *If your loved one decides to stay at home during the fragile years, make sure that the home is set up to accommodate them as they become less mobile and may need walkers or wheelchairs. There are certified "aging in place" specialists who can help you make the home safer and more accessible. Handrails in showers and bathrooms are just one feature you might add. Bathtubs with "doors" that allow easier access can be another smart move. Chair lifts for stairways or home elevators are also popular for aging family members.*
- *Medicare does not cover home care aides or most long-term care, except for doctor-prescribed nurses and therapy for limited periods.*
- *Some states have Medicaid waiver programs that provide for care in the home. Some even allow you to hire friends or*

> *relatives as caregivers. Check with local agencies like www.
> eldercare.acl.gov to see how it works in your area.*

- *If you hire a home care aide on your own, check references
  and background carefully. There are services that will hire
  and screen them for you. They charge fees that are usually
  well worth it.*

- *You can arrange for your parents to see therapists when it
  works best for them. For example, if your parent is receiving
  physical therapy, occupational therapy, and speech therapy,
  you can schedule them for different parts of the day to allow
  time for rest.*

Chapter Six

Caring for the Memory Impaired and Others with Special Challenges

I was visiting one of my clients with dementia when she screamed at me:

"You're fired! Get out of my house!"

This wasn't the first time this poor woman had turned on me, and I knew it was simply her impairment and confusion that triggered this outburst.

So, I went out the front door, waited outside for fifteen minutes, then went around and knocked on her back door.

She opened it and said, "Thank God you are here, I hated that other bitch."

"Oh yeah, she's awful, isn't she?" I replied.

Sometimes, you just have to find the humor in life, especially when you are dealing with aging parents with Alzheimer's and other forms of memory and cognitive impairment. They can be the most difficult, the most expensive, and the most heart-wrenching to care for; believe me I know.

Yet, many of the most rewarding moments I've experienced in my career have been with the same sort of clients, who can experience moments of sweetness and clarity between mood swings.

A favorite memory: I was visiting a ninety-four-year-old client whom I just loved. A pleasantly confused, tiny little lady with thick eyeglasses that made her beautiful eyes swim. She was on her huge couch, sinking into the cushions. I joined her so we could speak eye to eye.

I was there with her daughter because we were moving this woman out of her home and into assisted living. Her daughter was running around the house, doing last minute checks to make sure everything was packed.

"I'm ready to go," she said quietly.

I knew she wasn't talking about moving to the new community.

"Are you?" I responded. "That must be a good feeling for you."

"Yes, it is, I could go anytime," she replied.

We sat quietly watching her daughter rush about. She then said to me, "I don't know if she is ready for me to go."

She wanted to sign a "do not resuscitate" order as part of getting her legal paperwork organized. We had several conversations before she decided that no extraordinary measures should be taken if she had a medical emergency.

"Do you want your daughter to know how you feel?"

"Yes," she said.

I summoned her daughter from another room.

"Your mom wants to talk to you."

The harried daughter, who was worn out from caring for her mother and worrying about her, sat down. She was eager to get her mother moved so she could return to her job and life.

Nothing was said for a few seconds as we took in the importance of the moment. Finally, her mother looked at her and said, "I'm ready to go when the time comes."

The daughter burst into sobs and tears. We sat for a few more minutes, not rushing it, willing time to slow down.

That moment has stayed with me, and I hope the daughter has had the same experience. It is beautiful when a loved one has a moment of clarity like that. Those are the experiences that lift my heart and sustain me in my work.

Caring for a loved one with a memory impairment in a family home can be exhausting. Sometimes, family members become overwhelmed and lose track of the person they once loved. They forget that this fragile individual is still the same person who cared for them earlier in life, loved them, and helped them find their way to adulthood.

As I was writing this chapter, I met with a woman who wanted me to assess her mother, who was in a nursing home, and then recommend a care program for her. She wasn't sure if her mother needed to move into a special unit. Her mother had memory impairment and other cognitive issues, but she was generally compliant, though not very active.

The daughter asked her mother: "Would you join Amy and me for dinner?"

The mother did not respond. She no longer understood the concept of going to dinner together.

The daughter looked at me, not knowing what to do.

So, I stood up and put my arm out for her mother to latch on to. She stood up and we walked arm and arm into the dining room.

When we reached our table, the mother just stood there. So, I sat down. Seeing that, the mother sat down too.

At first, there was no conversation, but the daughter had told me that her mother loved to sing. So, I began singing. Softly, because I am not a great singer. I knew the mother liked a certain song with the lyrics, "Let me call you sweetheart." I sang that.

The mother joined in. Other residents seated around us joined in too. Once the meal came, there wasn't a lot more conversation, but I could tell the mother had enjoyed herself. By taking the lead, I took the pressure off her, and that was something she needed in that moment. When verbal communication goes, emotional or non-verbal communication steps in.

Knowing What They Need

For the purposes of this book, I use dementia as a catch-all name for a range of behaviors and symptoms that can include forgetfulness (usually short-term memory), difficulty processing information, and behavioral issues such as aggression and wandering. It is not a psychiatric illness, but the elder with dementia may exhibit what appear to be psychiatric problems. There are neurological issues in the brain that can cause a wide range of physical, mental, and emotional challenges.

In the more advanced stages, the patient may not be able to perform simple tasks like bathing or answering the telephone. They can experience confusion over basic things like the time of day, the month, year, and present location. Some undergo personality changes as well as hallucinations and delusions. Finding the right words to express themselves is also a big frustration.

Though Alzheimer's is the most common form of dementia, affecting one in ten people who are sixty-five or older, there are many varieties of memory impairments, which is itself a catch-all for any form of dementia.

It is also true that no two clients are alike. There is a general set of symptoms, behaviors, and approaches, but honestly, you cannot apply any one set of rules or recommendations to caring for all who have memory impairment and cognitive issues.

That fact is one of the reasons caring for someone with a memory impairment is so frustrating. Behaviors can change by the day, and a strategy that worked one day may not work the next. They are all unique in how they act and in how they respond. Some become quite mellow and sweet. Others can be belligerent and violent. And any one of them can swerve back and forth in that range.

The saying in my business is that if you've worked with one client with dementia, well, you've worked with one client with dementia—so don't expect the next one to act in the same way or to respond to the same approaches. To make it all the more challenging, there is no single test for it.

Common early signs are forgetfulness, losing track of time, or becoming lost in familiar places. More advanced dementia can adversely impact short-term memory, the ability to move about even at home, basic communication, ability to perform personal care, and understanding what is going on around you.

In the most advanced stages, the person with dementia may lose all awareness of time and place, lose mobility, fail to recognize loved ones, become aggressive, and be unable to manage personal care.

The older person with these symptoms may need to undergo a series of medical, cognitive, and lab tests. Nailing down just what form of impairment someone has can be even more difficult because symptoms can overlap. The standard list includes:

- Alzheimer's Disease
- Early-Onset Dementia
- Frontotemporal Dementia
- Lewy Body Dementia
- Mild Cognitive Impairment
- Mixed Dementia
- Parkinson's Disease Dementia
- Vascular Dementia

I won't try to describe all the forms and ranges of dementia here. My goal is to help you and your loved one once a diagnosis has been made. My job with this book and for all in my profession is to help families find ways to provide daily care in a safe setting, while managing the financial and emotional challenges that arise when an older person you care about has impairments that make independent living impossible.

Figuring out which form of dementia is afflicting your loved one can be a long, arduous process, and maybe the wrong thing to focus on because there is no cure for dementia in any form. I know it can be comforting to have a name and medical explanation for whatever is tormenting your parent, but even then, you still have the practical problems to contend with. Some want a diagnosis, especially if there is a genetic component that might mean they are at risk of developing the same diagnosis.

This was one of the points of a recent documentary, *Robin's Wish*, about the actor and comedian Robin Williams, who committed suicide while suffering from what was originally diagnosed as Parkinson's disease. An autopsy and study revealed three months after his death that he'd actually had a related but more challenging condition called Lewy body dementia.

I've heard this described as "the most common form of dementia that you've never heard of." In my business, however, we are all too familiar with this cruel affliction that attacks the brain and the body, causing havoc that includes hallucinations and paranoia as well as physical torment. It's also extremely difficult to treat and manage because the behaviors can be so erratic. No medications are effective in working with these behaviors.

There are support groups for nearly every form of memory and cognitive impairment, though I've found that many caregivers can become overwhelmed by them. I have heard many say they want help with handling the problem, but they don't want to sit around and talk about it.

Some listen to others and learn and feel supported; to others, it's overwhelming and they feel worse after a support group. It can be helpful to bond with others facing similar challenges, but I've known people to feel support groups are too stressful and draining.

Many are comforted knowing they are not alone, yet it can be overwhelming when others share the worst-case scenarios and the tremendous emotional and financial burdens they've borne. This is why many clients come to us, so we can help relieve and support them with our expertise, knowledge, and contacts.

A Word of Caution on Diagnosing Dementia

I will caution you that whenever someone calls me and says they think a loved one has dementia or Alzheimer's, I listen very carefully as they describe the symptoms. Sometimes it's critical to make certain of that diagnosis. In other cases, the behaviors are so challenging that some form of de-escalation has to occur first.

It can take months to get a firm diagnosis, and even then, the problem behaviors still have to be addressed. Those who work often with older individuals are always cautious and proceed slowly because we know that a sudden loss of memory in an aging individual can be due to a simple urinary tract infection that is easily treated, or due to delirium brought on by anesthesia if the elder has recently been hospitalized for surgery.

In the aging population, a urinary tract infection can trigger hallucinations, aggression, confusion, and distraught behavior that is often mistaken for early onset dementia. Years ago, I had a client admitted to a psychiatric facility, only to be diagnosed with a urinary tract infection. So, we urge families not to rush to judgment and to, if time allows, proceed with a very thorough medical and neuropsychological examination.

I had a client who had her seventy-eight-year-old father with clinical depression forcibly moved to a mental health behavioral center because he had become aggressive toward his caregivers after two weeks of confusion and lethargy. Interventions had not been successful.

A distraught family member called me for guidance on what to do with him. I knew the geriatric psychiatrist in charge of the psychiatric unit of the hospital, and he was one of the best in the region. The psychiatrist recommended that the man be admitted to the medical unit first. Soon after admission, they found he had a urinary tract infection on top of his clinical depression, which contributed to his sudden aggression.

They had to treat him for the urinary tract infection before addressing his severe depression. Then, they worked with him for two or three weeks and got him to a functional level before moving him into a retirement community that was affordable and provided meals. He's been there for two years as of this writing.

There can also be other causes for common dementia symptoms. For years now, there has been growing concern that when fragile older people are given anesthesia, they can have memory loss as well as confusion and even hallucinations. Many of us in the field often see that anesthesia can make a memory worse or, in some cases, seemingly cause a memory impairment.

One of my friends and consultants whom I will write more about later in the book, geriatric psycho-pharmacologist Lori Daiello, is conducting research in this area to determine how pervasive and long-lasting the impact can be.

If there has ever been a case of dementia in any form that was easy to manage, I'm not aware of it. Every client is different, and there is no treatment to "cure" the disease or reverse the brain damage. There are drugs that we are told can maintain a current memory or slow the decline to a degree and ease the symptoms, but even then, the medications do not work for everyone in the same way or to the same degree. It's been refreshing to see some of the work being done regarding exercise and socialization as preventive measures against dementia.

Financial Challenges of Care for Those with Dementia

For most families, the financial challenges are considerable when caring for a loved one with dementia. The average lifespan after being diagnosed with dementia is eight years. At first, the client often needs just a little bit of supervision. But as the dementia progresses, the individual needs more care and supervision.

Most families do not plan for the cost of assisted care, which is needed when the loved one is not yet dependent enough to move into a skilled nursing facility, where Medicaid offers coverage.

I will write about the public benefits availability in another chapter, but it's important to know that most states do not have a generous in-home or assisted care public benefit program.

One of the biggest gaps in our system is assisted care for older adults, and older adults with a memory impairment fit in this category for a lot of years. In addition, memory care is labor intensive and much more expensive.

According to several senior resource websites and the Care Management network, these were the monthly median costs of long-term care, assisted living, and nursing home care in 2020 in the US. It is important to remember geographical differences—with California and the Northeast United States generally having higher costs than the southern and midwestern states.

- *Home care: A paid non-medical home health aide is $23 per hour and $1,012 per week.*
- *Adult day services: $75 per day.*

- *Assisted living facilities: $4,051 per month or $48,612 per year. Ranging from $2,800 to $9,500 per month. In addition, fees can move upward from $1,000 to $2,500. Fees can be negotiated and broken into installments.*

- *Memory care in any community typically adds about $1,200 per month in additional costs.*

- *Private room in a nursing home: $280 per day or $102,200 per year.*

- *Semi-private room in a nursing home: $247 per day or $90,155 per year.*

Source: Genworth. Cost of Care Survey 2019: Median Cost Data Tables. Available at: https://www.genworth.com/aging-and-you/finances/cost-of-care.html

In Central Florida, where our operations are based, the average cost of memory care assisted living is closer to $6,000 a month, and that price can double in other areas of the country, particularly in the affluent regions of the Northeast and California.

Typically there is not a lot of state Medicaid funding available for assisted care, which includes care for those with memory and cognitive impairments, but each state is different. Many are surprised that room and board is not covered by Medicare. Medicare is insurance designed to pay for medical care, not for room and board and other daily expenses known as "maintenance care."

Running out of money before they die is one of the biggest fears of older adults. They tend to try to make it as long as they can without care, which frequently ends in a catastrophic event (most often a fall and a broken hip), and they are forced to receive help, sometimes in a more restrictive environment than they wanted.

It is an ironic truth that assistance is easier to get if you can prove that you are impoverished than if you have some limited financial resources. The cost of care is high, regardless of how much money you make. It is true that if your loved one runs out of money and lives in a nursing home, Medicaid will kick in and pay.

Take Care of the Caregiver, First

When funds are not available for nursing homes or other alternatives, we often see at least one child take on the role of care provider to an aging parent, which can put a lot of strain on families. The most worrisome situations arise when the spouse of a memory-impaired person serves as the full-time caregiver in the home. This can create an untenable situation in which the "well" spouse eventually is hospitalized due to the stress of caring for the one with the memory impairment.

It can be both heartwarming and scary to see a husband or wife caring for their spouse. Such devotion can have a high cost because of the high level of care required and the stress it generates. Often, the caregiving spouse will give up if the dependent spouse becomes incontinent.

I counsel the loved ones of those with dementia to take care of themselves first, but it often takes more than one conversation to help them understand the importance of that. Financial worries and guilt weigh on them. I worry about family caregivers, especially spouses and partners, as much or more than the clients themselves because no one is monitoring their physical and mental health in most cases.

There are scores of support groups online for those whose loved ones have Alzheimer's or dementia. Most communities also have a network of organizations, non-profits, and support groups that can help you take better care of yourself and the afflicted person. I would recommend hiring a care manager in the area to provide you with the resources available in the community, saving you time and mental stress. They can help you develop short- and long-term plans.

Most people aren't prepared for the sudden mental decline of a parent or loved one. Panic can set in quickly, and before you know it, you can feel over your head at a time when you need a clear head and a plan.

I once had a high-strung woman client—we'll call her Roselyn, which is not her real name. She hired me to oversee the care of her mother, who was in the very early stages of dementia. The mother was still mostly just pleasantly confused, but she was at a stage where she would ask the same questions over and over and tell the same stories repeatedly. The mother was happy, but Roselyn was coming unglued.

The daughter was stressed over her mother's condition even at that early stage. Roselyn was beating up her mother's caregiving team about getting her more and more therapy all the time. I finally staged an intervention of sorts.

Sometimes the work of a care manager is helping align the adult children with the reality of their parent's situation. Diplomacy is required. I told Roselyn:

"Your mother is so sweet and pleasant. She's doing fine. But your state of mind will give you a heart attack if you don't ease up, and then your mother won't have you looking after her interests anymore."

"There are counselors, therapy, education programs, and books that will help you come to terms with your mother's diagnosis," I told Roselyn. "It's normal to take her memory impairment behaviors personally, but you need tools to move through this very normal process."

Some of the stress was related to the cost of care. My team helped the mother secure Medicaid and VA benefits to pay for care for her and some counseling for Roselyn. As a result, Roselyn was able to enjoy more time with her mother. The daughter participated in programs offered by the mother's community. They found a great peace in knowing that the time they did have together wasn't fraught with fear, tension, or financial concerns.

Going with the Flow and Maybe Fibbing Now and Then

The children of aging parents with dementia often will fall into an understandable but misguided pattern of trying to "fix" their loved ones in hope that they can return to a normal life. They might correct the individual when they say something wrong or even chide them for memory failures or the inability to perform daily routines.

That approach never works. It can only lead to greater frustration and resentment. My advice for dealing effectively with those with Alzheimer's and other forms of dementia is this: embrace lying and fibbing and manipulating when necessary. The goal is to give those in the fragile years some peace of mind. If you find that your words escalate their frustration or aggression, simply stop talking.

Do not try to correct their behaviors or the things they say. If they have on two different types of shoes, go with it. If they are wearing two shirts or their pajamas are on backward, let it pass. Be comfortable with who they are in each moment, knowing their behavior can change dramatically at any time.

You have to experiment all the time with them to see what works. Your goal is to win a "yes" from them, to foster cooperation and trust. Now, that isn't always easy. For example, many of our clients with memory issues do not want caregivers or aides in the house with them.

To win them over, we find out what is important to them, whether it's really good home-cooked meals, clean sheets, help with tying their shoes, or just someone to listen to their stories. Then we have the caregiver provide those important services.

We train our caregivers to provide those desired things in abundance while winning the client over. It's not always easy. It doesn't always work. But most of the time our people have the skills necessary to win the trust of the client. This takes a lot of patience and emotional intelligence.

It's tough to accept someone into your home, especially if you are confused and feel vulnerable. As I mentioned earlier, I have been told by many older adults that admitting they need in-home care feels like a surrender or an admission that the end is near for them.

In my first year in practice, I went to do an assessment on an older woman who refused to talk to me. She would barely look at me. I asked her adult children to leave the room. Then, I asked her if she thought I was there to put her in a nursing home.

"Yes," she said.

She feared that I would make her move out of her home because her kids wanted the house for themselves. Once that was said, I asked her what type of help she would prefer. In the end, I helped bring a caregiver into the home to help with cooking, cleaning, and running errands. I also asked the children to stop interfering with the care at home, as it increased their mother's anxiety.

Some clients enjoy caregivers who talk to them, while others prefer their caregivers to be quieter. Often, it takes some time to find a good match by finding a home caregiver with the right personality and chemistry for the client.

Special Challenges

Those with memory impairment and mental challenges may experience hallucinations and paranoia, which may require a lot more patience and expertise. You have no doubt read or heard of once loving spouses who no longer recognize their loved ones. Often, the older person mistakes a child for a spouse, which can be unnerving. It's not unusual, either, for them to forget they are married and become enamored of someone else.

Probably the most publicized case of this occurring was with the husband of former Supreme Court Justice Sandra Day O'Connor. She retired as a justice in 2006 to focus on caring for her husband, John, who'd been a lawyer with a prestigious Washington, DC, firm.

She shared the story of his decline in many speeches and media interviews to advance understanding of Alzheimer's and its impact. In 2000, John O'Connor went to see a neurologist without telling her because he was having trouble remembering words and writing at work. Her husband's condition worsened after the diagnosis.

The couple sold their home and moved into a condominium initially because Mrs. O'Connor was afraid John would wander and get lost if there wasn't a doorman to stop him. After several months, her husband no longer recognized her, and she feared he would hurt himself without constant supervision. She then moved him into an Alzheimer's care facility in Phoenix.

There, he became attached to another woman. Mrs. O'Connor handled this wisely. When she found John sitting with his new friend and holding her hand, she would sit on the other side of him, holding his other hand.

Sadly, the former Supreme Court Justice was diagnosed with Alzheimer's herself in 2018, after she'd spent years as an advocate for her husband and others with the disease. She retired from public life at that point.

When a loved one has Alzheimer's or other forms of cognitive and memory impairment, you could do worse than follow Sandra O'Connor's approach and learn to be patient, going with the flow. My guidance is always to slow down everything, your lifestyle and your responses and reactions.

Taking It Slowly

I've had family members call me for help at the first sign of memory issues in a parent. They assume that the parent needs to move into an Alzheimer's care facility right away; as a matter of fact, often, family members want care to begin much faster than their parents. But, really, that isn't usually necessary or even desirable in the early stages of most forms of dementia.

The family members are concerned that they won't be able to give the proper care to the family member with dementia. They are often stressed out over the responsibility and challenges. When adult children are stressed out like that, we often suggest that the first step should be to get the parent into an assisted living facility and see how that goes, rather than moving straight into a more expensive memory impairment facility or unit.

Rapid changes in their living environment can make things worse for loved ones already struggling with physical, mental, and emotional challenges. They may become angry and hostile, feeling that they are being moved out of the home against their will. Imagine how you might feel if you lost your memory and one day woke up in a strange place. Really, sometimes not moving out of the home is the best solution for the elder, but the most stressful for the family.

I had one client tell me that with his memory impairment he woke up every day feeling like he was in a foreign country—and this guy was still living at home!

Over the years, I've heard it said that no one truly learns patience until they get married or until they have children. Those may be steps along the way, but I believe there is nothing more challenging than having a loved one with Alzheimer's or a similar form of dementia and cognitive impairment.

You have to have patience in abundance, as well as creativity and kindness. Aging parents with memory impairment may forget to bathe for weeks or change their clothes. I had one Alzheimer's client whose adult children gave up on trying to get her to wash her clothes. Instead, they'd buy her duplicate outfits of the same clothes she wore every day. They'd wait until she was out or asleep and then take her dirty and worn outfits, replacing them with the new clothing. She never seemed to notice.

Another client with severe memory impairment became highly dependent on her beloved dog as a constant companion. One day, her caregiver called me in a panic.

"Her dog died! She won't be able to handle it. What do I do?"

"Don't worry, I've got this," I said.

Then we went out and found a nearly identical dog, just about half the age of the deceased one, and switched them out. She never caught on.

I am not kidding when I say you have to be creative when a loved one has a memory impairment. My father had dementia in his later years. One day, he became very upset because he couldn't find the ignition key to start his wheelchair. There was no ignition key for his wheelchair, of course. He was confusing his car, which he was no longer allowed to drive, with his wheelchair.

Rather than trying to sort all that out with him in his confused state, I simply took a key off of my own key ring and pretended to turn his wheelchair on so we could ride around the nursing home. He thanked me, told me I was "brilliant," and immediately calmed down as we took a long lap around the facility.

Be Cautious about Hiring Home Care Workers

Many people hire part-time or full-time home care workers to help their impaired loved ones stay at home. That can be a wonderful solution if you can afford it and if you can find trustworthy people.

I always caution those with aging parents to do thorough background checks before hiring anyone to work in the home with them. There are predators who pose as caregivers who are skilled at winning the trust of and then stealing from vulnerable older people.

You have to be smarter than them. Companies like mine do very thorough background checks for any criminal records or other issues before sending aides into the homes of clients. There are far too many cases out there where a home care worker has gained access to an older person's bank accounts and credit cards and robbed them blind.

We were called in to help a ninety-seven-year-old woman who had hired a home aide without checking out her credentials or criminal background. When the woman's nephew, who was her guardian, went to visit, the aide would not let him into the house. He called his attorney, who called us.

This was one of those occasions when my job became more like a *Mission Impossible* operation. The aide, who'd somehow secured power of attorney for the woman, was obviously up to something. She wouldn't let anyone talk to the woman who'd hired her.

So, we waited for the aide to go to the grocery store. The nephew took his aunt to a hospital twelve miles away for evaluation. When the aide showed up at the hospital with her power of attorney papers, the aunt told the nurses she didn't want to have anything to do with her.

Her nephew had convinced her that the aide was taking her money. We later found that the aide had worked for several older relatives of the woman before discovering that she was the family member with some money. The aide then targeted her.

This is all too common. I've worked with one family whose older relative had hired a predatory caregiver who convinced the fragile older person to get married. Another con artist posing as a caregiver swindled $50,000 from the client to pay for her daughter's college. There are many examples of exploitation of the elderly, which is why we always advise people to be extremely careful in hiring home caregivers.

Sometimes, the caregiver isn't really a predator. Relationship boundaries in home care can easily get blurred. Sometimes exploitation happens because the elder feels sorry for the caregiver or just wants to help them. Keeping financial information out of the house protects the caregivers as well as the elder.

Finding a Place for the Challenging and Fragile Parent

As my father's memory and cognitive impairment progressed, he moved from living with me and my husband to assisted living and then into a nursing home. We never felt the need to put him in a special home or unit for the memory impaired, even though that was always an option if his condition reached the point where he needed highly specialized care.

I note this because many adult children assume that a parent diagnosed with Alzheimer's or a similar condition should be moved into a facility or unit that is designed for those with memory and cognitive impairments. Each case is different, of course, but I'm usually very cautious about making that big and expensive move right away. And, 50 percent of those eighty-five and over have some level of cognitive deficits—not all of them need specialized care.

The number of places that specialize in care for Alzheimer's patients has grown exponentially in recent years to serve the growing number of people afflicted with memory disorders. The demand is there, and so are the financial rewards for the owners of those highly profitable facilities.

At the same time, more and more assisted living and nursing care facilities have developed their own designated rooms or wings of rooms for the memory impaired. My initial preference in most cases is to keep fragile loved ones where they are most comfortable and at ease, even if they've been professionally diagnosed with dementia—as long as they are safe.

The operative word is *safe*, which usually means that there is someone with them at all times, or most of the time. This often applies to those with mild and even moderate cases. Someone in the care management field can help you sort out your many options according to the needs of your parent or loved one.

I've found that some clients in the early and moderate stages do just fine staying at home, especially if they can attend a cognitive fitness day care program from nine to five each day. This provides them with the stimulating environment recommended for them, and it also takes some of the burden off family members.

Many of our clients stay at home with mild to moderate dementia when they have the financial wherewithal and the risk is acceptable. The aides help with meals and nighttime routines, literally tucking the clients into bed.

For those who are more confused or have unmanageable behaviors (wandering out of the house or high levels of aggression), moving to a specialized community is the best strategy. Families may want to let the parents stay at home if that was their wish. It is true also that some older adults are more introverted and wouldn't adjust well to a communal style of living.

I have observed that many of our clients adjust very well in a specialized unit because the pressure to perform is over. Their behaviors and confusion are accepted as the norm, and they actually flourish in a community with trained caregivers, vibrant activities programs, and a community that is designed to allow them freedom of movement.

Alzheimer's units are typically for those who are aggressive, easily agitated, and difficult to deal with. They are at risk for escape or injury to themselves or others. The staff in these units are trained to handle these behaviors and try to support the person where they are as opposed to trying to get them to comply.

We were recently hired to help with a client who had memory and cognitive impairment but was living in a standard assisted living home. When our care manager went to assess him, she noted, and the staff confirmed, that he was spending a lot of time "stalking" around the front entrance of the facility.

We agreed that he appeared to be planning an escape, so we contacted his daughter and recommended that her father be moved to a more secure memory care facility. While we were arranging that, he made a break for it. The police were called to track him down and bring him back. He was then moved into a memory care unit, where he will remain until he is no longer at risk of another great escape.

Memory units and homes specializing in the care of residents with Alzheimer's and similar impairments also provide stimulating programming throughout the day. This is so helpful for those with a shortened attention span. This programming also helps maintain short-term memory recommended for those with moderate to severe symptoms.

The science on how to care for those with memory impairments has grown tremendously in the last ten years. A staff with special training for these residents can make a huge difference in the quality of their lives. They have expertise in dealing with their personality and mood changes, their anxieties and fears, and their need for stimulus throughout the day.

When you walk into a facility for residents with memory and cognitive impairment, you should see a lot of activity programming. Most of the good facilities will have programs at least twelve hours a day, including cooking classes, exercise programs like tai chi and range of motion workouts, as well as singalongs, music performances, art classes, and supervised outdoor walks.

The top-quality facilities will have stage-driven programs that meet the changing needs of residents as their impairments progress. Most have very brief attention spans, so the programs should be very engaging. If you walk into a facility and everyone is watching television or staring off into space, turn around and run. You want your loved one to be somewhere that keeps their neurons firing as much as possible.

When family members tour a facility, they should look for administrators experienced in specialized care. There are dementia-training certification programs for staff, and it is good to know that they've had that training, but you should observe how the administrators and staff interact and communicate with the residents and each other.

I always watch to see if staff members make the effort to put their eyes at the same level as those of residents they are talking to. That's an important thing for those in the fragile zone. You don't look down at them or up at them, you look them directly in the eyes in a non-intimidating, caring manner.

Most staff will make a point of knowing each resident's name and nickname and a bit about their background, but do the residents respond well to them? Feel free to ask staff members how they would respond if your loved one took a fall, or became agitated, or refused to take medications or participate in programs.

The layout and décor is also an important factor for those with Alzheimer's and similar challenges. For example, shiny floors are not a good thing. They shouldn't be slippery at all. And a black and white décor is also not recommended because it is too harsh, but you don't want overly bright and intense colors like reds, oranges, or purples because they are too stimulating. Calmer, softer colors like pale yellows and greens are considered better.

You want to come away from your tour of a facility feeling blown away by what you've observed and learned. There should be a lot of activity and efficiency as well as cleanliness and order. If residents and staff are just sitting around idle, that's not a good thing. If their interactions lack warmth or familiarity, that's a problem.

There are many very comforting, supportive, and safe places for your loved one with memory impairment, and I encourage you to keep looking until you find the best and most affordable facility for them.

Key Questions When Looking at Memory Units:

- Does the staff have training and experience with dementia patients? Where did they receive their training?
- What are the hours of activity programming for residents? Are these provided by staff employed by the community, or are the activities programs outsourced? Or a combination of both?
- What environmental support is provided by the community itself? During the tour, the staff should be pointing

out the environmental support built into the community including wall colors, outside walk areas, activity rooms. A rule of thumb: the more a facility resembles a home, the better.

- Medical facilities should be separated from living areas, hidden or discrete.

When Your Loved One is a Threat to Others

Finally, I want to address a subject that is rarely mentioned but presents substantial challenges. When an aging loved one is afflicted with memory and cognitive impairment, there can be huge shifts in mood and temperament. The person you know and love may undergo personality changes that are totally out of character. This includes violent behavior and aggressive sexual behavior as well.

Finding a place for someone with these challenges is extremely difficult, as you might imagine. We were involved in a case in which an eighty-three-year-old man with dementia got into trouble while visiting his wife in a nursing home.

This guy was wheelchair bound, had significant hearing loss, and wore thick-lensed glasses. He did not look like a threat to anyone. But an aide in his wife's nursing home reported that he was "physically inappropriate" with his wife's roommate during his visit.

The nursing home filed criminal charges, and the husband pleaded no contest to the charge. He thought that would be the end of it, but because he did not contest the charge, he was put on the registered sex offender list.

His daughter hired us to move him from his apartment into an assisted living community, leaving out the fact that he was on the registered sex offender list. When word got out that a registered sex offender was living in that community, all heck broke out. Television crews showed up in the lobby. People protested.

I had been hired by the couple's daughter to manage their care, so when the assisted living center called me wanting him moved to another facility, I called the daughter.

"I forgot to tell you he was a registered sex offender," she apologized. She then told me the story of how that had happened.

"Where can I find him a place?" she asked.

I managed to get him into another assisted living facility, but he was only there two months before the police were called. Someone had checked the local website for registered sex offenders and identified him as a threat.

The administrator of the senior living center was madder than a wet hen. They wanted the old guy out of there. Before I could intervene, they shipped him out to the hospital emergency room, which is one of the ploys care facilities use when they want to get rid of a problematic resident.

The facility claimed he was sexually inappropriate with a nurse and he was a "danger to himself or others," the legal mechanism that frees them from having to readmit him back into the facility.

The head of care management at the hospital called and told me the facility would not take him back. I knew this director well, so I said, "You and I will just have to figure this out together."

We finally found a good assisted living center that agreed to give him a chance. I convinced them that an octogenarian in a wheelchair who was nearly blind and hearing impaired was not all that big a threat to anyone. The administrator took precautions, and the confused old fellow did fine. He lived there for eighteen months without incident and passed away.

I have had far more aggressive clients with dementia, including another male who had a habit of grabbing nurses inappropriately. We managed to keep him from getting thrown out by adjusting his medications.

If an older person is judged to be a danger to others, a care facility can send them to the hospital for an involuntary psychiatric admission for seventy-two hours. If the dangerous behavior is stabilized, he can be freed after that period. I would recommend asking what was done to stabilize the person, and also pushing to extend the stay in order to have the person evaluated and treated.

You want to secure as much help as possible to prevent another involuntary admission, in case the problem wasn't fixed in the first place. If the behavior does not improve, a court hearing will be held in the holding facility or hospital to determine how long the stay should be extended.

I advise loved ones that if a parent is placed on involuntary psychiatric admission, they should remain calm and try not to over-react. Sometimes this is what is needed in order to become stable enough to live in a community setting. What you do not want to happen is multiple psychiatric admissions, which can make it nearly impossible to find a placement in a care community.

The psych unit may limit who your parent is allowed to speak to. It is usually limited to the POA and/or their designee. In the case of an involuntary psychiatric admission, you should make sure they have been medically cleared, eliminating medical conditions that might be causing the problem behaviors. Once any possible medical issues have been addressed, the psych unit can focus on the issues at hand and stabilize the individual without creating zombie-like behaviors.

Geriatric psychiatric units can be extremely helpful if the older loved one's behavior is unmanageable anywhere else. But, they are few and far between. Another challenge is the fact that difficult behaviors due to cognitive impairments don't meet the criteria for admission to most psychiatric units because dementia is not a psychiatric diagnosis.

To manage this situation, you can get help from a local geriatric psychiatrist. They can be found through the American Association for Geriatric Psychiatry's website: www.aagponline.org.

Keep in mind that getting an appointment with a geriatric psychiatrist may take weeks or months because there are not many of them out there. It's also true that nursing homes are forbidden by law from physically or chemically restraining residents unless the issues are well documented. They must reduce the restraints or show they have tried to reduce the restraints on a regular basis.

Some send such patients to the ER, but hospitals will blackball a nursing home that does that repeatedly. This issue in my opinion is the hardest situation for families to manage and for the elder to receive appropriate help.

If an elderly parent is acting out sexually, consider having a doctor prescribe estrogen, which diminishes the sex drive. This can be controversial, and some states do not allow it. But I have seen situations where it was used (with permission of course) temporarily and it worked. If it hadn't, the resident in the nursing home would have had nowhere to go.

Your Takeaway Tips:

- *Caring for a memory-impaired parent can be exhausting and emotionally draining. Do not isolate yourself. Tap into support groups or get professional guidance. Learn where you can find day care, practical guidance, the best doctors, and other resources.*

- *Work with a caregiver to teach them the best methods for communicating and handling your parent.*

- *Tell the caregiver about your parent's life to create a picture of your parent before the diagnosis.*

- *Early on, make sure you have power of attorney and access to their finances and important records.*

- *Don't argue with memory-impaired people. Don't correct them. Save your battles for when it really counts. The goal is to connect and provide for their peace of mind.*

- *Take a dementia training course with an instructor well-trained in dealing with dementia patients.*

- *Shorter, frequent visits are better than longer stays, and participating in activities with your parent can be enlightening and rewarding.*

- *Don't pressure them to understand anything or to accept reality. Don't ask questions that require answers. Adjust your approach if they become agitated. Remember they will have difficulty settling down if they become frustrated or agitated.*

- *Go with the flow until they can calm down. Understand that it takes them longer to adjust to new situations.*

- *It's a good idea to register your memory-impaired parent with the Alzheimer's Association and their Safe Return program*

> that provides ID cards and a nationwide photo database,
> especially if they are at risk for wandering.

- *The playlists of soothing music available on Pandora and other streaming music services are an inexpensive source of comfort and pleasure to many of our clients who sit for hours indoors or outdoors and listen to their favorite songs, enjoying the memories they stir.*

- *Going online to see old neighborhoods or take tours of loved museums, parks, and the like is fantastic fun for the elder and the caregiver.*

- *Do not keep credit cards, debit cards, banking information, or any financial information at the house once caregivers are helping.*

- *I advise clients to do exercises to maintain brain fitness rather than taking medications for keeping a memory intact.*

Chapter Seven

Pharmageddon: Prescriptions for Disaster

"*My dad is ninety years old and in a nursing home, but they want to kick him out because he is acting crazy, threatening people and grabbing women. I've called five other nursing homes, but no one will take him because he is so difficult to control.*"

I investigated this client's father and learned that he'd recently begun to show "bad behaviors" that often occur as dementia progresses, so the nursing home doctor prescribed medications to control mood and psychotic disorders. The meds seemed to only make matters worse, which is often the case with older people. This is especially true with those who have memory and thinking problems caused by Alzheimer's disease and other types of dementia.

As we grow older, our bodies and minds respond to medications differently than when we are younger and healthier and can effectively remove medications and their byproducts from the blood. As we age, our ability to break down and eliminate certain types of medications from the body slows. This is one of the reasons that older people should be prescribed lower doses of certain medications—this is particularly important with medications that affect the brain.

In addition, when an older patient has two or three or four doctors independently prescribing meds without consulting the others, the combination of different drugs can play havoc with the person's physical and mental health.

Just recently, I saw a new client whose daughter had to track her medication on an Excel spreadsheet. The woman was on sixteen medications. That is a problem!

I deal with this all the time with our clients, but the potential for serious problems caused by the interaction of multiple medications is often overlooked. Failing to recognize these problems can result in falls and broken bones, memory problems, frequent doctor's visits, hospital admissions, and possibly death.

Too often, their families and even their physicians write off odd behaviors as the results of dementia, or they attribute physical problems to "aging," but many times the unrecognized problem may be a serious interaction between prescribed medications—often in combination with over-the-counter meds and supplements.

We call this the "Pharmageddon problem." Because we've dealt with it so often, we always check a client's list of medications before considering a dementia diagnosis. We know the most common drug interactions that can trigger dementia-like symptoms, but if the case is more complicated, we call in our own Sherlock Holmes (or Dr. House), who has superpowers of detection when it comes to the properties and interactions of prescription and all other types of drugs.

Our favorite pharma-detective, Dr. Lori Daiello, is a rare bird with an unusual title. She is one of a small group of pharmacists who specialize in geriatric psychopharmacology, and her sub-specialty is working with older people who are taking a mix of medications that can adversely affect their brains and their physical health.

In simpler terms, Dr. Daiello is an expert at sorting out the interactions of prescription drugs and their impact on elderly patients. For example, she once helped me with a client who was taking seventy different prescription medications and suffering all sorts of ill effects that had to be sorted out to determine what was causing her symptoms.

Dr. Daiello starts her detective work by studying all of a client's physical and mental health issues, along with the medications the client has been taking. The next step is recommending step-by-step changes in the medication list to the doctor. Working together, a new plan is developed that often leads to a smaller list of medications that help stabilize the person, so they receive the care they need without further complications.

These pharmacist experts can be life-savers when the "cure" is worse than the disease. They really are like private investigators who gather evidence while trying to figure out medical mysteries. The victims are older people, many of them in the fragile zone, who are having mental, physical, or emotional challenges.

Too Many Meds Prescribed by Too Many Physicians

We call in Dr. Daiello when a client is exhibiting challenging behaviors such as hallucinations, out of control aggression, or sexually inappropriate actions. We trust her expertise in evaluating our clients and helping us determine whether their behaviors are a result of medication issues. We check to see if the person might be on the wrong medications or taking a combination of medications that is triggering the problem. She has also found certain supplements that can cause problems on their own or in combination with other medications or supplements.

"Usually, the clients referred to me are at the far end of the spectrum as far as their medical issues," she says. "They may be taking as many as twenty plus prescriptions or more, over the counter medications and supplements too."

The patients may suffer a wide range of mental, emotional, and physical problems that cannot be attributed to the usual causes by their physicians. Many case investigations are complicated by the fact that older patients are reluctant to share with their doctors what is in their medicine cabinets, especially if they are buying supplements like CBD oil, herbal medicines, or mega-vitamins online without first consulting with their doctors.

The reasons for this reluctance can be because they don't want to tell their doctor the drugs are making them sicker, or because they feel guilty for taking so many pills, or even because they are taking a bunch of supplements to defy the "highfalutin" medical establishment and pharmaceutical industry. Of course, sometimes, they just can't remember what they are taking on a daily basis.

That's what makes Dr. Daiello's job so interesting. Every patient is a new mystery.

Supplement Warning

In some cases, we have discovered that an older person having issues was being given a harmful supplement by a well-intentioned but misinformed adult child or friend. The individual really did not know what the supplement was or the dangers they can cause when interacting with other medications.

We had a person in assisted living whose blood pressure went sky-high, and at first the medical staff couldn't figure out why. Then we discovered that her son had decided the woman's antidepressant wasn't working well enough, so he gave her St. John's wort, a supplement that is often advertised as an antidepressant or mood regulator.

The problem is that St. John's wort can cause bad interactions with some medications, including the prescribed hypertension medications this woman was already taking.

When we asked her how much St. John's wort she was taking, the woman said, "It depends on how upset my husband makes me, but maybe two to four pills a day."

St. John's wort speeds up the breakdown of certain antihypertensive drugs, so the more of it she took, the higher her blood pressure went. She was in danger of having a stroke because her son was playing doctor. He meant well, but he didn't know what he didn't know.

There are dangers also with some supplements, depending on country of origin, that may be contaminated with heavy metals like lead or other toxins that you don't want to be ingesting. Supplements from China or other countries taken as holistic medical treatments have been found to contain medications that are prescription drugs in the US but not in other countries.

If you're concerned about whether your supplements might be potentially harmful or ineffective substances, Dr. Daiello recommends the website ConsumerLab.com, an independent organization that reports the results of their tests on many types of supplements on their website, which can be accessed through an inexpensive subscription service. They also review supplements, including those with CBD oil, and they will tell you if a supplement sample doesn't match up with the ingredients listed on the label.

Dr. Daiello also suggests that older people take their supplement bottles with them when they meet with their physicians, so they can ask them about any potential problems the supplements might have when taken with their prescribed meds or over-the-counter meds.

Expertise on Drug Interactions Is Difficult to Find

In truth, even many family physicians fail to catch problems related to drug interaction because generally they don't have much expertise in that area. Pharmacology may not be covered in depth in medical school programs for family doctors. After medical school, some may find that their fast-paced practices don't leave much time for reading medical journals and may come to rely on medication updates and information from the pharmaceutical industry and their sales representatives. As a result, in my opinion, family physicians often don't have the latest information about potentially dangerous drug interactions.

Consult with your family doctors, but also be ready to serve as your own best advocate. You have to be diplomatic but firm. Most physicians don't like to be challenged, but they should be open to your questions and concerns. I wouldn't recommend you start a conversation with, "You know, I read online that this blood pressure medicine you prescribed...."

However, an older friend recently told me that in a discussion with friends who also were taking blood pressure medication, he learned that the medication that his doctor prescribed for him was more powerful because it was designed mostly for those who'd suffered heart palpitations or arrhythmia—neither of which he'd experienced.

When he questioned his doctor about it, the doctor said, "But I thought you'd had those issues?" Now, this doctor had been his physician for a long time, but the doctor clearly had it wrong. He admitted the mistake and changed the prescription to a more appropriate blood pressure medicine for this patient.

Dr. Daiello and I encourage our aging clients and their family members to talk to their doctors regularly about *all* of their medications, prescribed and over-the-counter, as well as *all* of their vitamins, herbal remedies, diet pills, and stimulants—including Red Bull and other "energy booster" drinks and pills. Many contain high levels of caffeine and even ephedrine, which can cause serious problems for people with heart conditions.

If your physician prescribes a new drug, make a point to ask whether the new medication might react in adverse ways with any others you are taking. If your doctor brushes you off, let them know you are concerned, especially if you start feeling poorly or having memory, concentration, or sleeping problems after taking the drug.

As We Age, Our Bodies Respond Differently to Medications

As children and young adults, we all tend to respond to medications in similar ways, unless we have serious health issues. But as we get older, the aging process affects our organ and brain function as well as nearly every other aspect of our bodies. If you have played heavy contact sports like football, boxing, and wrestling, you may have suffered concussions and other injuries that altered your brain and perhaps caused deterioration of your shoulders, elbows, wrists, knees, and ankles.

That is why older people generally can't rely as much on the drug interaction software programs at their pharmacies. We need to keep ourselves safe as we age.

Here are some basic guidelines for doing that with your medications and anything else you take to fight off aging, sleeplessness, or depression, or to soothe weary bones and worn joints.

A Seven-Point Prescription for Safer, Saner Use of Medications

1. Find a friendly pharmacist.

The most accessible source of information on this issue is your local pharmacists who specialize in medications for older clients, particularly those who work with nursing homes and assisted living centers. They are likely more aware of what to look out for when an older person is having unusual symptoms that can't be easily explained.

We recommend also that older people and their caregivers get most of their prescribed and over-the-counter medications at one local pharmacy, so the staff there can check records and monitor your meds for any potentially harmful drug interactions. Their record-keeping software usually posts alerts automatically, however, that software does not always take into account the age of the customer, which can make a big difference in how they respond to many drugs and drug interactions.

Having a pharmacist who knows you, your prescriptions, and your health issues can save your life, so this is advice to take to heart. More than most family doctors, they receive extensive training on the benefits and possible dangers of medications, so pharmacists may be the first to alert you to potential problems caused by your medications or their interactions.

If you are in a nursing home, don't be afraid to have a trustworthy pharmacist check on the dosages being given to you by the nursing home drug dispenser. Often, they don't have a great deal of training in medication interactions in older adults, so they may not be monitoring your prescriptions carefully.

Now, these days it is common for many older people to get their medications from online pharmacies where you can't have personal interaction with pharmacists. There are resources available, however, if you or an aging loved one have questions about medication interactions as a possible concern.

You might begin your search for answers with the American Society of Consultant Pharmacists website, which will help you locate a qualified senior care pharmacist in your area (www.ascp. com). Senior care pharmacists are specialists in understanding the effects of medications on aging bodies and minds and can help you with a complete review of your medications. Senior care pharmacists are trained to recognize medication side effects disguised as health problems and can confer with your doctor about taking action to eliminate these issues, such as lowering some medication dosages, switching to a safer medication, or even stopping those medications that are no longer needed.

2. Start low and go slow on any new prescriptions.

Most physicians have had this message burned into their brains since med school, but it doesn't hurt to remind them that you are aware of it too. Starting new medications at low dosages and taking it slowly will help you determine if the drug is helping—or simply causing side effects.

However, in some cases, that message should be changed to, "Start low and go slow—but go!" What happens all too frequently is that for some medications, the low starting dose is supposed to be increased gradually to a higher but effective dose. If this step is forgotten, then the medication may work partially—or not at all.

I've had clients who told their doctors that their medication wasn't working, so the doctor simply prescribed another med without stopping the original one. The clients end up taking both, and as a result, they end up having bad side effects, which may involve a hospital stay.

Dr. Daiello notes that as we age, our brain is much more sensitive to effects of sedating medications, in particular. So, if you were taking a Xanax prescription of four milligrams a day in your forties and fifties, it's highly unlikely that you can take the same dose into your seventies and eighties without side effects.

"I had an older relative in her eighties with mild memory problems," Dr. Daiello said. "Her doctor had been prescribing her medications to treat anxiety and depression for a long time, without lowering the dosages as recommended for older people. When I brought it up, the doctor did not agree to a plan to gradually lower the dosages of the medications that were worsening her memory function. She then visited a neurologist specializing in geriatric issues for a second opinion, who ultimately convinced her doctor that she was overmedicated."

3. Be aware of the danger when mixing meds and supplements.

One of the issues we run into with older people is known as the "prescription cascade." This occurs when someone takes two medications that cause a health issue, which results in another medication being prescribed to treat that issue. Too often, this results in additional prescriptions to treat new side effects created by the previous medications. This is how our clients can end up with large numbers of prescription bottles filling their medicine cabinets.

Sometimes the issue isn't two prescribed medications. It might be a prescription med interacting with a supplement of some kind. We have had clients who are taking warfarin to prevent blood clots have unexpected and serious bleeding issues if they also take supplements that are blood thinners, such as turmeric (curcumin).

Even aspirin and certain antibiotics can interact with warfarin and can pose a danger when combined with turmeric supplements. When certain medications or supplements interact with warfarin, the result can be severe and uncontrolled bleeding—and even death. People who must take warfarin should always consult with their doctor before changing their other medications.

Nonsteroidal anti-inflammatory drugs (often called NSAIDs), such as Advil (ibuprofen), can worsen kidney problems or hypertension, sometimes causing blood pressure to rise to dangerous levels.

I once asked Dr. Daiello to consult on a client who was taking galantamine for mild memory impairment. Galantamine, used to treat the symptoms of Alzheimer's disease, increases a brain chemical, called acetylcholine, needed for forming new memories. It is believed that this drug can help ease some effects of Alzheimer's, though it is not a cure by any means.

This client was upset because he didn't think the galantamine was working well enough, so he bought a "super cognitive" supplement at the local natural foods market. We tested it and found that it contained a Chinese drug very similar to galantamine. So, he was essentially taking twice as much of the medication than he'd been prescribed. As a result, he was suffering from diarrhea and headaches, which ended when he stopped double-dosing.

4. Keep in mind that pain is often not diagnosed properly in older patients.

There has been a lot of discussion in recent years about the over-prescribing of so-called "painkiller" drugs, but Dr. Daiello and I are at least equally, if not more, concerned about the undertreatment and underdiagnosing of pain in our older and fragile clients.

Among people with memory loss, we have found this to be a significant contributor to several cases in which fragile older clients have become violent or combative, hitting, pushing, and otherwise mistreating caregivers and family members. When older people are in pain, they don't want to be put in a bathtub or touched at all.

Too often, this irritability and aggressive or hostile behavior is diagnosed as related to their memory or cognitive impairment rather than a physical cause, like severe pain. So, instead of investigating what might be causing their pain, the doctors, nurses, or caregivers may increase sedative or other psychoactive medication. These powerful medications do absolutely nothing to relieve pain.

This often happens in nursing homes, where the tendency is to assume aggressive behavior is related to a diagnosis of dementia rather than actual physical pain. The attitude of the physician or caregiver is frequently, "Well, they aren't complaining about pain."

But older people with cognitive impairments often don't complain about pain because they don't understand the source of it or don't have the words to explain it. Instead, they push people away because they are hurting and don't want to be touched.

I received a call related to this issue that involved a married couple, both in their eighties, who lived together in an assisted living facility. The staff said the husband had become combative and uncooperative with them. They'd issued a forty-five-day eviction notice to throw him out. They said the wife could stay but the husband had to go.

At the request of their daughter, I asked the administrator to give us some time to sort out what was going on. They had been married for sixty years, and the daughter wanted to keep them together if possible.

The husband was acting out of character, so Dr. Daiello took a look at his meds. She saw that he was prescribed a statin for heart disease. The medication was prescribed to prevent strokes and reduce his cholesterol.

Statins have been known to cause leg pain in older people. His wife was in a wheelchair and relied on him to push her around all day. He had complained that all of the walking was painful for him.

"My legs are killing me," he'd said.

I found that the husband had been taking the statin for years at the same dosage level.

"Too often, we see that doctors prescribe a medication, and a patient takes it for a decade or so without anyone on his medical team asking whether the dosage is still appropriate for his age," said Dr. Daiello.

This case was not unusual. It happens all the time. The husband hadn't associated his leg cramps and pain with the drug that he'd been taking for so long, so he hadn't mentioned it to his doctor. He was also on digoxin to control his heart rhythm, and, because of his age, his kidneys weren't flushing it out adequately, so his blood level was very high. Digoxin can cause confusion in older patients, among other side effects.

For the husband, Dr. Daiello recommended stopping several of his medications that were no longer necessary and reducing the dosage of others, which helped to greatly reduce his pain and combativeness so that he could stay in the community with his wife.

5. Reduce meds and improve quality of life as you age.

We remind our clients all the time that the guidelines used by physicians for prescribing many common medications may be based on drug studies that mostly include people younger than sixty, with very few people in their seventies, eighties, and older. Because of the general lack of information on the effects of medications in older people, their doctors and caregivers need to constantly monitor the effectiveness of their medications and any potential side effects for those in the fragile years.

A study on statins prescribed for eighty-year-old patients found that taking them off the medication had no greater adverse effect than leaving them on it, according to a report in the Journal of the American Medical Association (JAMA).

Both Dr. Daiello and I are advocates of the "deprescribing movement" that calls for a more thoughtful and proactive approach with the goal of "doing no harm" to the most vulnerable older people. This involves taking those in their fragile years off meds that may no longer be appropriate or necessary and may, in fact, cause more harm than good.

The deprescription movement is very big in Australia and Canada and growing in the United States, which, hopefully, will make physicians and pharmacists more aware of the harmful effects that many medications can have on fragile older people.

6. Make the most of Medicare wellness exams.

Older Americans with Medicare medical insurance are eligible for free, annual "wellness" visits to their physicians. The goal is to update your medical information and make a preventative plan to keep you healthy. The physician can also perform a cognitive impairment assessment to check for any signs of early-stage memory impairment. There may be co-payments and other fees for any tests that are ordered as a result of the exam.

I encourage my clients to make the most of these exams. Prepare for them by making a list of concerns and questions, and take along a list of your medications, vitamins, and supplements along with their dosages and expiration dates.

Then talk though the list of meds with your doctor to make sure your dosage is appropriate for your age and conditions. Your goal should be to reduce the meds you take and their dosage as much as can safely be done. Remember, this shouldn't just be an assessment of your prescription drugs. It should be an accounting to determine whether they are working and still the best option for you.

Too often, physicians don't take time to really talk with their patients in these exams, so you have to make a point to share information and encourage discussion. This should be a "personalized" plan aimed at preventing major illnesses, so get personal with your doctor. The physician should ask you to fill out a questionnaire, called a "Health Risk Assessment," as part of this visit. It should include a review of your medical and family history as well as an update of your doctors and prescriptions. Your doctor's staff will also record your height, weight, blood pressure, and other routine measurements.

Ask your physician to provide you an assessment of any risks and treatment options, recommendations for staying healthy, and any preventative shots or screenings you should schedule. Keep in mind that you need to be your own best advocate. I tell my clients that no one in the fragile years should go alone to physician appointments. They need advocates to help them and the doctors understand exactly what challenges exist and how to address them. The advocate can help prevent medical issues resulting from miscommunications and lack of support.

7. Protect your mind and your memory.

Dr. Daiello had a seventy-two-year-old patient with common medical problems including trouble sleeping, high blood pressure, chronic pain, and a history of fibromyalgia, causing discomfort and aching. Upon investigating, she discovered the woman was taking a strong dose of amitriptyline, an older antidepressant that was adversely impacting her memory, to the point that she had abnormally low scores on memory tests.

It was determined that her memory problems were entirely the result of high dosages of the medication she was on. Once Dr. Daiello had the dosage cut back on the antidepressant and on an anti-anxiety medication, the women tested in the normal memory range. The change was profound. She returned to normal once her meds were adjusted.

Dr. Daiello tells me that at least 50 percent of those who come to the memory disorder clinic where she is affiliated are found to be taking meds that adversely affect their ability to think and remember things clearly.

She has put together a list of those drugs that can affect and accelerate memory loss, including certain over-the-counter medications commonly prescribed for bladder control or enlarged prostates.

Also, one of the early symptoms in people developing memory problems is that their sleeping involves far less of the important deep sleep stage. Now, in their younger years, they might have taken Tylenol PM or other anticholinergic sleep aids to get more rest. But the more you take those types of medications, the more they can adversely affect your memory.

Even when you are young, this is true, but they can be a more serious problem as you enter the fragile years.

Your Takeaway Tips:

- *If your parent has a psychiatric condition, make sure you bring their meds to the hospital and closely monitor how quickly the staff secures those meds. Let the hospital know that you will give your parent the meds on schedule if for some reason the hospital cannot.*

- *As we age, our bodies respond differently to medications due to changes in hormones, metabolism, blood flow, and a host of other factors. The children of aging parents should monitor and regularly evaluate what over-the-counter and prescription drugs and what combinations of those drugs they are taking and the impact on their physical, mental, and emotional health.*

- *Make sure all of your parent's doctors know ALL of the medications they are taking. Doctors are notorious for not talking to each other about shared patients.*

- *Keep an updated list of all of your parent's medications in case they need to go to the hospital, where it will be critical information for the ER doctors and other staff members.*

- *Older people can suffer adverse side effects from common drugs including sleeping pills, pain medications, antihistamines, and muscle relaxants.*

- *If your parent is in a nursing home or assisted living facility, keep close tabs on what medications they are being given. It is not uncommon for staff to overmedicate residents to control their behavior or simply by mistake. You are supposed to be notified of all changes, but this does not always happen.*

Chapter Eight

Stopping Repeated Hospitalizations and Overtreatment

Ernie was eighty-seven years old, homeless, and living in a car until a Good Samaritan gave him enough money to pay for a few nights in a hotel. But after a couple days, Ernie fell down in his room and could not get up. The hotel manager alerted the local Adult Protective Services agency, which came to the rescue.

Social workers found Ernie a room in an assisted living center, but it became apparent that he preferred living in his car. He was a classic curmudgeon. Cantankerous to the core, Ernie gave the staff fits.

Nurses, aides, and administrators were always on alert around him because Ernie was known to throw the contents of his bedpan at anyone within range. He was an octogenarian terror.

In other words, Ernie was my kind of client. I happened to visit his domain while working with another client. While there, I heard the stories of Ernie's rampages. They described him as an angry old resident who refused to settle down.

I have a reputation for finding ways to work with challenging residents, so I accepted the Ernie challenge when a staff member asked me to find some way to restore peace and order. I don't have a bag of tricks; I just listen and show empathy. I enjoy talking with older adults about their lives. They tend to be more honest about their emotions at that stage of life.

Ernie and I hit it off right away. Like my father, he was a salesman from the Midwest. I asked him about his life, and he opened up to me. When he seemed comfortable, I asked him about his issues with the staff.

"They tell me that you throw your urine at them, Ernie. Why are you so mad at them?"

"If you were in this much pain, you would be mad too!" he said.

"What hurts you so much?" I asked.

"My leg," he said.

I checked his chart. Ernie had complained about leg pain, but the staff couldn't find a source for it. As a result, they weren't giving him any pain meds. I talked to the medical staff, and they worked with his doctor to figure out the source of the pain and to create an appropriate pain relief program.

Ernie mellowed out a bit after that; at least there was no more urine tossing.

Peace returned to the assisted living center.

I checked on him now and then, and Ernie seemed to settle down. He was still grouchy, but that seemed to be his baseline mood. Then one day when I went to his room, he was not there. The staff said he'd gone to the hospital after a fall and never returned.

Ernie had no one in his life—no family or friends. I worried about him. I'd had clients who became lost in the system after being sent by assisted living centers to the emergency room. This is a knee-jerk response all too often by nursing homes as well as assisted living centers. The administrators don't have the medical staff to treat serious medical problems, but they are also very wary of being sued, so they ship residents to the nearest ER whenever there are any medical or behavioral issues, no matter how slight.

Residents like Ernie sometimes are not allowed to return to their centers, so the hospitals ship them out to any place that has a bed for them. This can result in a disastrous series of events for an older person. They often end up in unfamiliar places and feel abandoned.

I have seen too many clients transferred back and forth repeatedly between care facilities and hospitals. I've also seen far too many unnecessary procedures done by hospitals on older patients. Hospitals and surgeons profit from operating on patients, and they are trained to fix and cure, even if there are substantial risks that the older person's quality of life could be adversely affected.

I couldn't get Ernie off my mind; we had bonded. I didn't know where he was, but I had to find him. Ernie didn't know it, but he'd just become my adopted client.

It only took a few days to track him down. Ernie was in a hospital's intensive care unit. He was on a feeding tube, oxygen, and another machine I did not recognize.

He smiled when he saw me, which was a relief. He was rational, another good sign.

"What can I help you with?" I asked him.

"Can you get me a glass of milk?" he replied.

I requested milk from a nurse, who seemed to resent my request.

"No!" she yelled. "He can't have anything by mouth. Doctor's orders."

I tried to explain this to Ernie.

"You might aspirate and choke if you drink anything," I said.

"I don't give a goddamn what happens; I want a glass of milk," he replied.

I went back to the nurse, trying to mediate.

"Ernie wants a glass of milk and doesn't care about the doctor's order," I said. "Maybe you could find the doctor while I go find him a glass of milk."

The nurse looked at me like I was a bad rash.

I knew this situation would escalate, but Ernie was frustrated, thirsty, and wanted to get out of there. I was Team Ernie. So, I bought a small carton of milk and took it back up to his room. I was opening the milk carton for him when his doctor walked in.

Busted!

"Will I be in trouble if I give him this milk?" I asked.

"Yes," said the doctor.

"He can't drink or eat anything because he is at risk for aspirating," the doctor said.

I am not a nurse, let me be clear, but I have heard this a lot over the years. The truth is that hospitals are mostly worried about their legal liability—and the bottom line. They make money by treating patients. If an older person wants palliative care, they don't receive it in the hospital. The hospital's first priority is not an older person's quality of life. It is to administer treatment.

It is simply easier and safer for them to control and monitor Ernie's eating and drinking by sticking a tube in him.

I was in full advocate mode. Ernie really wanted some milk, and he wanted out of there. I wanted Ernie to get what he wanted.

"Are you Ernie's designated decision maker?" the doctor asked.

"Ernie, do you want me to make decisions on your behalf?" I inquired.

"Yes," he said.

"Well, doctor, I guess I am!" I said.

The doctor looked relieved and gave me a big grin.

"I will have the staff get the paperwork together," he said.

The doctor walked out, and I gave the old guy some milk.

The next day, the medical team unplugged Ernie from all of the medical devices while I made some calls to get him transferred to a nice nursing home.

It was a heartwarming and satisfying feeling to see Ernie adjust well to his new home. Oh, he was still yelling at the staff, grumpy as ever, but he stopped throwing things and received no more aggressive medical interventions.

Ernie lived for four years in that facility. He did make one brief trip to the ER, but I'll share more on that later.

A Broken System for Treating Older People

If your loved one is in a nursing home, be prepared to step in if the staff suddenly decides to ship them to an emergency room. Preventing a hospitalization is tough, but it can be done. I tell my clients to avoid it if at all possible.

Nursing homes send patients to the ER for any medical event, even seemingly minor issues. The reasons for this are complex and frustrating; nursing homes are highly regulated and frequently sued.

Emotions run high when these transfers occur, with frantic family members trying to do what is best for loved ones in assisted living and nursing homes. The sad reality is that the most frequent result of these hospitalizations is a decline in health for the older person, not an improvement. And everyone who works with older residents knows this, including the nursing home staff and the hospital staff.

Usually, the families are the last to know a transfer is happening. The systems (government regulations and corporate procedures) do not make it easy to prevent these episodes. The administrators and staff usually do not tell families the truth about the high risk involved in a hospitalization.

Family members tend to hold out hope that a trip to the hospital will bring their loved one "back to normal." This is not usually the case, unfortunately. Once older patients in fragile health are admitted to a hospital, they are likely to be subjected to all sorts of tests and procedures that may well make them even more fragile and dependent. All too often, I've seen clients in their eighties subjected to heart valve replacements and other procedures that leave them dependent.

This is not just my opinion; this problem of overtreatment of older patients has been well documented by experts in the field. A veteran cardiologist recently told me that he is constantly in conflict with his fellow doctors over this issue.

"I work in a large cardiology practice, and I've been treated like a pariah by my partners because I often fight against doing surgeries such as heart valve replacements on people over seventy-five years old," he told me. "I argue that we have to treat older people in a more holistic manner, focusing on the quality of life they want, rather than subjecting them to tests, procedures, and surgeries that may prolong their lives but leave them bedridden, unable to communicate, and miserable."

As I've noted, when older patients leave the hospital, it is often extremely difficult to find nursing homes or rehab centers that will take them if they need to stay long term, as they often do. Even when these frail patients do find a bed somewhere, they can end up being transferred back and forth from the hospital to the nursing home.

They tend to decline in health each time, creating havoc and stress, with no improvement in their quality of life. I'm often hired by the adult children of parents who've fallen down this rabbit hole. They are in reactive mode. They have busy lives with jobs, and many have children of their own, and suddenly they have the added responsibilities and challenges of increasingly fragile parents.

You can stand firm and be clear in these situations. It is okay to advocate for your loved one rather than follow the dictates of nursing homes and hospital staff who may have other priorities. Most of them will understand and appreciate what you are trying to do.

I know that isn't always easy because the caregivers and medical professionals say things that will scare you. They will tell you that if certain procedures aren't done, your loved one could suffer or experience a premature or painful death.

This information doesn't get balanced with what the downside is for the suggested medical procedure. And, if asked the question, "What are the downsides to the procedure?" medical staff aren't forthcoming most of the time. The truth is, since there are no clinical trials on older adults for most procedures and treatments, no one knows for sure what the downsides are.

I have heard medical staff tell patients' families that insurance wouldn't cover their stay if they didn't follow the hospital's plan. It's difficult at times for facility staff to keep their values to themselves. This plays upon your guilt and your lack of knowledge about the reality of your loved one's situation.

Freeing Ernie

My friend Ernie offered an example of these issues four years after I stepped in to be his advocate. By then, Ernie was ninety-one but still hanging in there. An independent ol' cuss, he had a tendency to overestimate his abilities. He'd stand up unassisted despite warnings from the staff.

Then he'd take off walking and, often, he'd take a fall. Ernie did not break any bones, but he tended to topple over. I know this because the nursing home staff called me repeatedly, demanding that I allow him to be sent to the ER because he'd fallen, again.

I'd always ask if he'd incurred any broken bones or other serious injury. And when they said he had not, I'd tell them to make him comfortable and leave him in his room. They stopped fighting me after about six months of this battling.

When Ernie did begin to decline dramatically, we put him in hospice care. He had become increasingly confused. He no longer understood that he had a catheter, which he had previously come to accept. He began yanking it out, and they wanted to hospitalize him to put it back in because he was tough to handle.

Ernie still hated going to the hospital, and he fought like hell when they tried to put him in the ambulance. He had a strong faith and often said he was ready to meet his maker, but not in a hospital.

At one point, an ER doctor called me and said they couldn't get the catheter in for Ernie, so they wanted to admit him to the hospital for a urology consult to resolve the issue of his catheter. I didn't want to see the old guy put through a bunch of tests and procedures that would only infuriate him.

I informed the ER doctor that Ernie was on hospice care and did not want to be hospitalized.

"Please return him to the nursing home hospice," I said.

There was a long silence on his end.

"We need to get his catheter in," he insisted.

"Or what?" I said.

"He will die without it."

Time to play hard ball.

"Ernie has been prepared to die for a long time. He loves his nursing home family. He's been clear for a long time in saying he doesn't want to die in the hospital, and he doesn't want a lot of procedures done to prolong his life. So, send him back, please," I said.

The ER doctor actually sounded relieved.

"Well, he has made it very clear that he doesn't want to stay here," he said.

We both had a laugh at that.

The ER doctor had to follow hospital protocol, but he seemed to understand that there was really no reason to keep Ernie in the hospital and put him through a bunch of tests that surely would be ordered by the urologist. And, somehow, they were able to get the catheter back in him, and he was sent home.

Once again, the nursing home called and said they wanted to send him to the ER.

I refused to allow it.

"He is nearing the end now, and he doesn't want to die in the hospital, so let's just make him as comfortable as we can in his room," I said.

The staff rallied around him, keeping him company almost around the clock. I brought my dog Stevie in for a final visit because Ernie loved him. Stevie laid for a long time on the old guy's stomach.

Ernie died eight days later, surrounded by people who'd come to care about him. I know that's how he would have wanted to go.

A System Based on Profit

I don't blame the nursing staff and ER doctors for following procedures with Ernie. They are caught in a capitalized health care system that doesn't easily support a person's wishes for comfort measures.

There are very good books focused on this issue, including *Overtreated* by Shannon Brownlee. They make it clear that it is very difficult to go up against a system that is set up to treat even fragile older patients aggressively.

The nursing home sends fragile residents to the hospital because their system almost requires it. The hospital receives them and tries to treat them because that is how they earn high levels of compensation.

Everyone is afraid of being sued, and as a result, patients are often shuffled back and forth until they end up dying in the last place they'd have wanted to be.

Once aging individuals experience a fall, a stroke, a heart attack, or another event that threatens their independence and weakens them, they can easily go into a spiraling decline. Perhaps their greatest challenge is avoiding stressful hospitalizations for treatments that all too often are unnecessary and, in fact, often severely degrade their quality of life in their final years.

Nursing homes, assisted living centers, and hospitals all have their own complex rules and regulations—and they can be bewildering. Determining what is covered and not covered by Medicare, Medicaid, private insurance, and VA benefits can also be quite challenging in these situations.

The adult children or others responsible for the aging person's care can easily become overwhelmed with these repeated hospitalizations. Complex insurance and financial reimbursement mechanisms can send adult children over the edge.

Family members are often frantic, overwhelmed, and distressed when they come to care managers like me with concerns about an aging parent in the middle of a medical crisis. Our first bit of advice is to take deep breaths and hit the pause button.

Our philosophy is: "When in doubt, buy time." We tell our clients that most fast decisions are the wrong decisions. So, the first step is to slow the decision making down so that each decision is hopefully a permanent, appropriate one.

We have developed effective tactics for doing this, especially when medical professionals are pushing for high-risk tests and treatments that frequently cause more harm than good, or when hospitals want to discharge aging patients with no safe place to go. There are actually key phrases (found in the Takeaway Tips) you can use to legally halt the discharge of an older person from a hospital or nursing home so that you can buy more time. For example: If you tell the discharge staff that "We have no safe place to send them at this time," they must give you time to find one.

That is why there is no need to make rushed decisions in most cases, despite what surgeons or hospital or nursing home staff might be claiming. In all cases, your decisions should be guided by what your parent wants, given all of the factors in play.

Hospitals and doctors are trained to prolong life, and it is their instinctive response to do whatever they can for their patients. Your responsibility, however, is to ask whether your parent would want to prolong life if it meant not being able to eat, walk, stand, or go to the bathroom ever again.

In my opinion, the easier decisions are when life support or ventilators come into the conversation. I hear people say, "Don't ever hook me up to anything." It's the more subtle issues that are not discussed, like the loss of function that can occur as a result of the test or a procedure. As I noted earlier, no studies have ever been done on hospital procedures for people over eighty. They are referred to as "evidence free."

When you advocate for an older person who has entered the fragile years, you have to deal with complicated health care issues, financial concerns, and a baffling multilayered insurance system. And then there are the emotional factors.

Time and again, the grown children of my clients tell me, "If she dies, at least I know that I made sure they did everything they could for her."

Those feelings are understandable and quite common. Yet, too often, we don't take into consideration what the elder person wants at the end of life in practical terms. Polls and studies show that typically 80 percent of the population prefers to die at home, not at a hospital or care facility. And studies have also shown that 80 percent of people over sixty-five die in hospitals, not at home.

On top of that, the risks of medical complications from infection, surgeries, and exposure to bacteria and viruses is high when a fragile older person makes repeated trips to the hospital and back.

That is why, when my clients desire support, I am aggressive in my efforts to limit trips to the ER and hospitals. I prefer to keep them out of the health care system altogether if that is possible. And often, it is.

My client's desires are my guide—not the hospital's desires, or the doctor's, or the nursing home's. Often, ER doctors and nursing home staffers are relieved when care managers step in as an advocate and say: "My client doesn't want to go to the hospital again, she wants to go on hospice care where she can spend her final days in peace."

Hospitals and nursing home staffers are locked into default responses by concerns about being sued and the steep regulations they have to manage if they don't take every measure to protect a patient or to prolong life.

When I was a health care administrator it was common in the industry to hear threats of lawsuits from families under stress and frustrated with the care their loved ones were receiving. I think care managers who understand all aspects of the situation can be strong advocates who protect the interest of the clients first. We know how to win those battles.

For example, while they won't often tell you this, nursing homes can treat a dehydrated patient with IV and antibiotics under a physician's directions, so there are options aside from shipping residents out to the ER time after time. You just have to know the right questions to ask. You can also be very clear on your parents' wishes to avoid being sent to the hospital for specific reasons such as shortness of breath or even altered mental status or falling out of bed.

Examples of questions to ask: When a nursing home wants to transfer a client to a hospital, we ask if the procedure can be done at the nursing home. If the nursing home says they cannot do the procedure, I ask if I can sign a document that frees the nursing home from liability when I decline the transfer.

This doesn't always work, but over time, the facility staff will learn that it requires a lot more of their time on the phone or in person if they send your loved one on an unnecessary hospital trip. Most of the time, nursing home administrators become more accepting of this, though they may not like it.

Emotional Issues

The adult child of a parent in the fragile years tends to want to do everything possible to prolong the life of the parent. It's difficult to follow the values of the parent when it conflicts with the desires of the child. It's particularly challenging because most care facilities will support the notion of prolonging life.

Those in the care management and advocacy business are trained to have "professional courage," so we can make the decisions that follow the desires of the older person. It is emotionally challenging to do that, which is understandable, but there comes a time when the desires of the parent should come first.

Most people do not want to be kept alive if there is no meaningful interaction with loved ones. If the older person has to be on pain medications that make communication impossible or difficult, there may be no sense for them in prolonging life.

That can be a very difficult decision, to be sure. A lot of people focus on obtaining a Do Not Resuscitate order, which to me is an easier decision to make than whether to put a parent on a medication to stimulate their appetite when they are in a nursing home. If a parent has lost the capacity to decide these issues, stepping in can be even more difficult.

Imagine yourself as the older person nearing the end of life. What would you want for yourself? Would you want your life prolonged by extraordinary measures if the procedures left you unable to communicate or interact with loved ones?

Would you want your life prolonged by more subtle measures? Appetite enhancers, high calorie drinks, special diets that would allow you to swallow and digest? (Have you seen a pureed meal? I have had many clients over the years say if that's all I can eat, I'd rather not.)

Now, what about your parents? Have they expressed feelings one way or the other in the past about what they perceive to be life-prolonging measures?

You will need an attorney to draw up the legal documents for health care decisions. There are complicated medical issues as well. An attorney specializing in issues for the elderly told me years ago that she preferred to have her clients work with a care manager who fully understands the situations they might face when an older loved one is in the medical system. Care managers and elder attorneys in combination are the ideal partnership to guide elders in this time of life.

As much as we want this to be a clear-cut decision, it is usually more complicated. Some family members may want to honor a parent's wishes for no extraordinary measures. Others may advocate that the doctors do all they can to prolong life. Sometimes the risk levels of procedures aren't at all clear, which makes it all the more difficult.

When you have a loved one in a care facility, your goal is to make it clear to all of the staff—and reinforced in the person's medical records—that you want to be called *before* they send your family member to the hospital if that is your loved one's preference. Repeat it over and over in care plan meetings and communication with the nurses and administrators about your position. Depending on what state you live in, the relationship that you develop, and the staff's tolerance for your going against the grain, this may or may not prevent an unnecessary hospitalization.

Your Takeaway Tips:

- *Be aware that nursing homes and assisted living centers will respond to most of your loved one's medical issues by sending them to the ER. That is their default procedure, but you can prevent some admissions by re-training staff, using your state's additional Avoid Hospitalization language, and in many cases simply refusing to allow the transfer.*

- *You can let the facility know from the beginning that your care plan procedure is to keep your parent out of the hospital unless it is absolutely necessary. During your admission meetings with the facility administrators, make it clear that you want it on the medical record that your loved one is not to be sent to the ER without your consent. Tell them: "Call me before you call*

911." *This does not guarantee they won't ever be sent out, but it might prevent a trip or two.*

- *Consider placing your parent on hospice care at the nursing home or assisted living facility. That tells staff that your loved one does not want to go to the hospital for life-sustaining treatments. When someone is on hospice status, a hospice physician or nurse oversees care. Hospice care is a Medicare benefit, so there will be no bill for hospice services.*

- *Educate yourself about portable medical orders (previously known as Physician Orders for Life-Sustaining Treatment, or POLST) in your state and how they might be used to help support your parent's fragile years decision making.*

- *Communicate clearly to the nursing home or assisted living staff what your parent's preferred course of action is in seeking or not seeking medical treatment. Some may have readily gone to the doctor. Others may have avoided doctors and hospitals with a passion. Some have no qualms about taking multiple medications. Others may prefer holistic treatments or no meds at all. Let them know the preferences of your loved one; although they should call you before any change in medication, that doesn't always happen. Tell staff at every opportunity to contact you before making any changes to medications for your parent.*

- *Develop relationships with nursing home and assisted living staffers. Take an interest in them and show gratitude and appreciation wherever you can. Tell them about your parent's life and personality. I have worked with many career caregivers who have devoted their lives to the older person and don't receive positive emotional support as often as they deserve it.*

- *Any time a doctor recommends surgery or treatment on your fragile loved one by claiming a high rate of successful outcomes, be very wary. There have been no scientifically valid clinical studies on any group of elders seventy-five or over.*
- *Ambulance drivers are required to take a patient to the nearest receiving facility. We have successfully made requests to transfer to a hospital deemed more appropriate for the presenting medical problem. It pays to ask the question. If your parent is taken to the hospital, make sure the hospital formally admits them. Ask the question: Has my parent been admitted, or are they on observation status? There is no financial reimbursement for rehabilitation in a skilled nursing facility if you were on observation status at the hospital. If you are not satisfied with the hospital your parent is in, you can transfer them to another hospital.*
- *Be aware that the hospital begins planning for the discharge of your fragile parent on the day of admission.*
- *You can delay discharge from the hospital for at least twenty-four to seventy-two hours by appealing the discharge decision.*
- *Do not let your parent be discharged from any facility after 5 p.m. or on a weekend. I promise, you will avoid chaos by following this tip.*
- *Understand that a hospital discharge planner works for the hospital's best interest, not for your parent's best interests.*
- *If your parent moves from a hospital to a skilled nursing facility (nursing home) and is too ill to begin therapy, you can delay therapy treatments for up to thirty days so your parent can regain strength. This is also true if a parent goes home from the hospital and needs therapy.*

- *Avoid sticker shock by asking about costs for transportation leaving the hospital or facility. Medicare reimburses for medically necessary transportation only. Trips leaving a medical facility are not deemed necessary, and it is NOT covered by insurance, costing hundreds of dollars.*

Chapter Nine

Finding Your Way through the Maze of Health Care Insurance and VA Benefits

After many active years managing a large bed and breakfast with her husband, Miriam fell down a stairway and broke her hip at the age of seventy-eight. Though she had claimed that she wanted to slow down and work less, Miriam had continued running the B&B and doing most of the housework.

Breaking her hip ended that career, marking her entry into the fragile years and a complex financial and health care maze. Fragile older people and their loved ones must make critical decisions not only about finding a safe place to live, but also about medical care needs, health insurance coverage, and finding financial resources to pay for what is not covered by Medicare.

Miriam entered the hospital on a Medicare Advantage plan. Once she recovered, she needed to go to a rehab center for physical therapy. The hospital provided her with a list of facilities. She and her adult daughter checked the ratings of the rehab centers on the list, and they were not impressed.

"There is not much of a selection here, and, from what we've seen, these are all low-rated facilities," the daughter told me when she came in for a consultation.

"This is something I deal with often," I told her.

"Rehab centers and nursing homes do not like working with Medicare Advantage clients because Medicare Advantage Plans are HMOs. They incentivize medical professionals to authorize *fewer* treatments," I told her. "As a result, those patients aren't very profitable for the rehab centers, so they prefer to treat those with traditional Medicare plans with supplemental insurance that typically pays for more treatments."

In my experience, clients with Medicare HMO plans often have to fight like crazy to get the care they need. Their treatments have to be "pre-authorized" by the HMO case manager for Medicare Advantage, who often denies the treatments that rehab directors want for their patients. This is a problem for older patients who need more therapy to become stronger so they can return to at least some level of independence.

In addition, if you are chronically ill and older and want to have a quality of life and get stronger through physical therapy, you have to fight to get it. Those who have the HMO plans usually don't have access to the best physicians or medical providers because the top-notch medical providers don't want to deal with Medicare Advantage Plans. The doctors want to control the treatments their patients get, and the HMOs are incentivized to authorize fewer treatments.

I think the Medicare Advantage HMOs have hidden costs passed on to family members because someone, whether it is the older person or their adult children or a professional care manager, has to spend hours and hours on the phone trying to help them get the best possible care while fighting the HMO. The hidden costs include taking time off work, the costs of hiring a professional to figure it all out, and the cost incurred for dependent care that could have been prevented had more therapy been provided—to say nothing of the emotional cost and stress of wondering if you are making the right decisions.

Now, on the other hand, you also have to watch out with traditional Medicare with a supplemental plan because there are risks that the client will be overtreated and given unnecessary tests or medical procedures because those are more profitable for the medical providers.

Again, every older person needs an advocate with their best interests in mind, whether it's an adult child, a friend, or a professional care manager hired for that job. It is a cruel fact that as we enter the fragile years, we are confronted with some of the most challenging decisions of our lives at a time when we often are in a physically and emotionally compromised state.

Too often, older people enter their fragile years and find themselves thrown into an unfamiliar world with its own language and byzantine, ever-changing rules and regulations. In many cases, their adult children are called upon to help them manage their Medicare and prescription drug plan. Those loved ones often find it challenging to figure out what is covered and what must be paid out of pocket.

The bombardment of questions can be overwhelming and the complexity of the answers simply maddening:

- *What is the best Medicare insurance plan available to me?*

- *The best drug plans?*
- *What levels of care are provided?*
- *Will they pay for a live-in aide? Assisted living? Nursing homes?*
- *If the doctor says I need a hip replacement, do I really want to go through that at this age? What happens if I say no? Will the anesthesia make me permanently confused after surgery?*
- *Where will I get the money to pay for everything not covered by my insurance?*
- *Am I eligible for Medicaid?*
- *Veteran's benefits?*
- *What does my long-term care insurance cover?*

Adding to the challenge is the fact that these decisions frequently need to be made quickly—clients in the hospital often are given only a few hours' notice before they are to be discharged. Skilled nursing facilities might give you a few days. There are ways to buy time, but no one in the facility will teach you what those ways are. I will provide suggestions on how to do that.

I've spent much of my career helping clients and their families answer those questions. As a professional care manager and former nursing home administrator, I don't always have all the answers, but I know where to find trustworthy sources for the information they seek.

Yes, it is extremely complicated. Honestly, stepping into this maze can be pure torture, but in this chapter, I will offer guidance to help you find your way. And I will provide you with key points and tips—the same tools I use on behalf of clients—so you will be less intimidated and better able to understand how to manage this unfamiliar territory that includes Medicare, Medicare Advantage Plans

(HMO coverage), Medicare Supplemental insurance, Medicaid, Long-Term Care Insurance, and VA benefits.

Introduction to Medicare

Medicare is the federal insurance program for those who are over sixty-five or disabled. It is funded by the Social Security Administration and administered by the Centers for Medicare Services (CMS). The program started in 1966.

It is a fee-for-service program with three parts: A, which is free, B and D with premiums. With B there is a premium normally deducted from your SS check. The premium increases annually with the 2021 premium now at $148.50. It is income based, and the premium increases for those who make over $87,000 filing singly and $174,000 filing jointly. The coverage is 80 percent with a 20 percent deductible which can be paid for by a supplemental plan through a private insurance company.

Medicare D is drug coverage, with an average monthly premium of $39 and a discounted cost for the drugs. It is also deducted from your Social Security check, typically. Open enrollment is in the fall, and it is highly recommended that you evaluate your drug plan coverage every year. We have seen significant changes in coverage in all of the D plans every year.

During Medicare's annual open enrollment each fall, you can change from traditional Medicare to a Medicare Advantage Plan and vice versa with no penalty or time without coverage. The change in coverage takes effect Jan. 1. The caveat here is that you may not be able to purchase supplemental insurance if a disqualifying event has occurred preventing eligibility for two years.

We have been asked by clients whether they should purchase supplemental insurance. Acknowledging that purchasing insurance is a very personal decision and some people are more risk averse than others, the most significant reason to purchase supplemental insurance is to mitigate the costs incurred with the 20 percent co-pay.

Keep in mind, there is no cap on the out-of-pocket costs with the 20 percent, so if a significant medical event occurs, you could be out thousands of dollars. Supplemental insurance can be purchased with a pre-existing condition with no penalty in the first six months of eligibility for Medicare. This is called a "guaranteed issue." After the six months, insurance companies can deny coverage. I tell clients there is also a little known supplemental plan that has $2,000 cap coverage, and once you pay that, the company pays the rest.

Medicare Advantage Plans are an "all in one" alternative to traditional Medicare. They combine Medicare A, B, and D into one plan, variously called Medicare Advantage Plan, Plan C, HMO, or a Medicare PPO. They frequently offer additional benefits like vision, hearing, or dental care. Both the cost and the offered benefits, such as dental care or visual care, may change annually. The list of health care providers, such as doctors, labs, and x-ray services, may also change from year to year.

The primary care physician is paid by the insurance company, and he pays everyone he refers to. Physicians have preferred specialists who are in their particular group. If there is a specialist you would like to see, and that specialist isn't in your primary care doctor's "pod," the doctor has the power to refuse your request for a specific specialist. Enrollees are federally prohibited to see a specialist without authorization unless it is for emergency care.

Advantage plans may have lower out of pocket costs, but not always. They usually have low deductibles but require co-payment fees for treatment or visits.

No. 1: Beware of not-so-advantageous Advantage Plans.

As I've noted previously, many nursing homes, rehab centers, and medical providers in assisted living facilities do not work with patients who have Medicare Advantage Plans. Keep that in mind when signing up for coverage.

The Medicare Advantage Plan is often pitched at "Free Medicare Seminars" held in steakhouses and senior apartment complex meeting rooms, as well as in relentless television and radio commercials, aggravating phone calls, and online advertising.

There are also predatory insurance agents who call older adults and convince them to change from traditional Medicare to a Medicare Advantage Plan without their families knowing and often without them fully understanding the downside to the change.

One of my colleagues worked with a woman who, during open enrollment, changed Medicare Advantage Plans three times due to a predatory insurance agent. The commissions are higher for insurance agents with the Medicare Advantage Plans than with supplemental insurance.

The more common PPOs allow you to see any health care provider in the insurance company's network without a referral, even specialists. Chances are your physician is in these larger networks. PPOs tend to be more flexible but slightly higher in cost than most HMOs.

Many older people are drawn to the lower cost of the HMO plans, but I've had far too many clients come to realize that these plans are not as flexible, nor are they as widely accepted as traditional Medicare.

I worked with a woman who had broken her leg and was in rehab with a Medicare Advantage Plan. She received two weeks of therapy under her Medicare Advantage Plan. We disenrolled her from the plan while in the facility. When the month ended and she was back on traditional Medicare, she received two more weeks of therapy.

There is a very good reason that insurance agents hype Medicare Advantage Plans. They make more money selling a Medicare Advantage Plan than supplemental insurance. However, Medicare Advantage HMOs really offer you *less* health care flexibility.

I've represented many clients who felt trapped in these HMO plans. The good news is that you or your loved one can bail out of Medicare Advantage Plans during open enrollment (in the fall of every year). And there are other times you can disenroll.

No. 2: Understanding Medicare and Medicare Advantage Plans

1. One of these escape opportunities for Medicare Advantage Plans can come if you are residing in a skilled nursing facility, even if you are staying only short-term. There are what are called "special exception" disenrollment periods. There may be a waiting period for a supplemental plan.

2. Understand that medical providers profit more when treating an older adult who has traditional Medicare and less

when a patient has a Medicare Advantage Plan. While Medicare with supplemental coverage covers all medical expenses (less a small deductible), it is important to remember that it is a fee-for-service program. Medical providers are paid a set amount for each scan, treatment, and surgery. For them, it is volume-based revenue.

If someone comes into a hospital for a medical issue, the hospital makes more money the more tests and treatment they provide. They are paid by volume. It is a traditional, capital-based plan, which gives rise to many ethical questions such as: *Does a ninety-one-year-old fragile older person with severe dementia at the end of life really need or want a pacemaker, considering all of the complications that could arise?* Chances are, no one at the hospital will try to talk you out of it or give you other alternatives because that's how they make their money, and because there is a fear of litigation.

The HMO model for Medicare Advantage supplemental is "capitated," meaning that the providing companies get paid a certain amount per year, per enrollee. Their business model means the *fewer* medical tests and procedures done for a client, the more money they make. Their profits increase when their clients get less care.

Medicare Advantage Plans may appear to cost less than traditional plans, but they are less flexible and not as widely accepted. There also will be charges for co-insurance that can run quite high when receiving care in a rehab center. The supposed attraction for an older person on an HMO is the perception, which is often false, that it is less expensive insurance.

The client pays a Part B premium, and drug coverage is provided. So, they save $200 a month in supplemental, or the co-pay at the doctor's office, which is not covered if you don't have supplemental insurance. Then the question that I have for clients considering Medicare Advantage is whether they are in, or are approaching, the fragile years. It has higher co-pays for hospitalizations and treatment such as chemotherapy.

The Advantage Plan also may not cover the twenty days of rehab in a skilled nursing facility. Do they have any chronic conditions? Also, does that extra $200 a month make a real difference for you? Clients in their eighties may need assisted living, and paying $200 for Medicare supplemental may seem like more of a burden. I advise them to consider their options every year, based on their needs and resources.

No. 3: Your Medicare policy covers "up to 100 days" in a rehab center, but 100 days is the maximum.

Let's say your mother breaks her hip, has it replaced, and then goes into rehab. You look at their Medicare policy and conclude, "My mom has 100 days in the rehab center covered, so I don't have to worry about where she goes next until the end of that period."

We hear that all the time, and then we have to tell the adult child that they've read the coverage *incorrectly*. The Medicare coverage is "*up to* 100 days." That's the max. The average length of stay in a rehab center under Medicare is between four and six weeks. If the fragile parent isn't showing steady improvement at that point, a discharge notice is issued, with usually a three-day notice, and discharge papers will be filed. When that happens, you are on three-day's notice to find a place to go if going home is not an option.

No. 4: Medicare does not cover medical care outside the US.

If you plan to leave the US for any length of time, call your medical insurer and find out what your options are. These can change, so always call for an update. You don't want to fall ill while overseas and have to pay for your medical expenses out of pocket. There are many nightmare tales of this happening, and you don't want to be one of them.

No. 5: Medicare clients often misunderstand what is covered for home health care.

Yes, you can get a home health care aide, but it is always short term and more of what we call the "drive by bath." If you are receiving therapy at home, you get a bath aide. When therapy ends, the bath aide stops. Medicare doesn't pay for live-in or part-time aides on a routine basis. This is called custodial or maintenance coverage.

The biggest expense for older people is the cost of assisted care, whether at home or in an assisted living facility. Often, these clients need just a little bit of help to stay independent, and nobody pays for that.

Medicaid will pay for custodial care in a nursing home, but only if the individual has less than $2,000 in assets and depends on help for critical things like bathing, dressing, going to the bathroom, and other major "activities of daily living" (ADL). There is

Medicaid coverage providing help in assisted living facilities or at home, and this varies widely state to state. In most states, if there is help available under Medicaid, it is not a lot of help, and there are usually waiting lists before care can be provided.

No. 6: Do not overlook possible veteran's benefits that may be available.

Many who have served in the US armed forces, or been married to someone who has served, are eligible for a little-known benefit through the Veteran's Administration. This benefit is not easy to access, like a lot of other VA benefits, a fact often reported in news media.

As I explained earlier, my father was among those who derived substantial financial assistance after I discovered he was eligible for the "Veteran's Aid and Attendance benefit," which will pay for a qualified veteran's or surviving spouse's out of pocket medical expenses, which includes assisted care whether in a facility or at home.

Many veterans are also eligible for a program that can help pay for their long-term nursing home care. When I was helping him through the financial and insurance maze, I realized he had never collected his Aid and Attendance benefit from the VA.

This is a pension that pays up to $1,936 for veterans, $1,239 for surviving spouses, and $3,032 a month tax free to veterans and their surviving spouses. To qualify, the veteran must be over sixty-five and have served at least ninety days of active duty with at least one day during war time.

The veteran must show financial need by having $129,400 or less in assets, and they must already be paying for certain care like bathing or help with going to the bathroom to be eligible. There is a three year "look back period," which refers to the government's right to examine your financial records to ensure you did not make any illegal transfers of funds in order to secure public benefits.

There are many ways men and women who have served our country can get help in their fragile years from the US Department of Veterans Affairs. But the rules and regulations for collecting VA benefits are so complex that many vets simply give up in frustration.

This benefit can be life-changing for those living in a community or receiving money for in-home care. It is frustrating that the medical and financial criteria for eligibility is extremely difficult to track down. The VA prohibits veterans or their surviving spouses from paying someone to file for these benefits, and many in the VA system are confoundingly touchy about this.

My contention is that you can hire professionals to file for your Medicaid benefits and to file your taxes, so why aren't you allowed to hire help when dealing with complex VA benefits? It's strange but true, and a real sore point with me because so many people come to us for help in dealing with the VA, which seems to relish withholding important information and creating complex regulations.

We have spoken with many people over the years who have made countless phone calls and emails with the VA and could not find consistent information regarding this benefit. Hopefully this section will provide some clarity on how to secure this benefit.

There is no income limit for this benefit, rather, to the degree the medical expenses as defined by the VA (for hands on care) reduce your monthly income, the benefit amount will replace the amount spent on hands-on care. For current information go to the Veterans Administration website va.gov or to my own Orourkeandassociates.com.

In Florida, the VA benefit can be used in conjunction with the Medicaid program in assisted living and at home. You might want to contact a care manager to determine if this is possible in the state in which you reside. Paying for assisted care is often the most difficult, as Medicaid in many states has minimal or no coverage until you get to the nursing home.

Assisted living administrators are usually grateful to learn a resident qualifies for this benefit, especially if they are faced with having to evict a resident because of inability to pay. I love educating people about these financial programs. It always makes me sad when a client comes to us facing eviction, especially when this eviction could have been prevented if they'd only known the rules of the game.

I met with a client the other day whose facility staff did not know there was a waiting list in Florida for assisted living Medicaid. His mother was down to her last $10,000, and he was faced with having to move her to a much less expensive home and a shared room. If the staff had told him to get her on the waiting list a year earlier, she could have received Medicaid benefits and continued to live in the community.

I have also experienced the joy of sharing good news with families that their loved one qualifies for the benefit and that they can stay in the facility in which they reside, or they may be able to afford to move into a community they didn't think they could afford.

My final thoughts to families would be to make inquiries about how Public Benefits and Insurance works long before you think you need to. This doesn't necessarily require your parent's involvement, but it will be one less thing you have to absorb when your parent starts to decline. There is so much more choice in care when planning has been done ahead of time.

Your Takeaway Tips:

- *Beware of not-so-advantageous Advantage Plans.*
- *Understand that medical providers profit when a patient has traditional Medicare with a supplemental plan, while the Medicare Advantage HMO profits more when clients get less treatment.*
- *Medicare Advantage HMOs may appear to cost less, but they are less flexible and not as widely accepted.*
- *Your Medicare policy covers "up to 100 days" in a rehab center, but rarely does an older person receive 100 days of coverage.*
- *Medicare does not cover medical care outside the US. Be sure to purchase travel insurance.*
- *Medicare doesn't pay for live-in caregiving OR maintenance care.*
- *Do not overlook possible veteran's benefits that may be available.*

Chapter Ten

Providing End of Life Care with Compassion and Grace

Sharon was a fragile older woman with severe Alzheimer's residing in a nursing home. Her adult children hired me to manage her care. When I visited her in the nursing home, I could see that she was nearing her final hours. No one in the nursing home had communicated with the family that she was dying.

She was curled up in a fetal position, sleeping most of the time, and unable to use the bathroom. She could no longer communicate because of her advanced dementia. She was hardly eating anything at all.

Her kids were understandably shaken by this news. It was gut-wrenching to have to tell them, even though I was doing what they had hired me to do in monitoring her condition and managing her care.

I suggested that they begin receiving hospice care in the nursing home which would allow her to die naturally, without any potential hospital admissions or inappropriate treatments to prolong her life. The nursing home communicated to me that although hospice would be involved, her physician would handle her treatment as well as the hospice physician.

As Sharon's advocate, I had an issue with the doctor's care at that point. My client was diabetic, and even though she was nearing death, the doctor was still giving her insulin and checking her sugar levels. That could be considered a life-prolonging measure, which typically is not done in hospice care.

The nursing home physician and facility staff were adamant about continuing this treatment, which was unsettling as my client's family were clear that their mother did not want any life-prolonging measures if she was clearly at the end of her life.

Why is it so hard to die in a nursing home? Facilities follow rigid federal rules. They are afraid of being sued. Could their administrators be suffering from compassion fatigue and fail to even recognize when someone is dying? Often, they cite "ethical issues," but it is really about avoiding lawsuits.

I asked Sharon's family whether they were okay with that, given her declining health. This was one of those very difficult conversations and decisions. I took some flak from the nursing home administrator for even bringing it up, but, again, I was hired to manage her care and ask the tough questions.

I talked with Sharon's children at length and informed them that, typically, families do not want their loved ones to be given life-prolonging medical treatment when they are in hospice care.

But, they decided that they were not ready to stop her insulin treatments. It was their choice, and even though I didn't agree with it, I certainly understood. There are many emotions that come into play in these moments.

Sharon remained in hospice care, getting her insulin treatments, for one month before she passed away. If the family had stopped the insulin treatments, Sharon likely would not have lived for four weeks. There were concerns that she would experience pain if her insulin treatments were stopped, but the doctor could have administered drugs to eliminate any pain.

The issue for me, in this case, was that an outside party brought these issues to light, and not the facility staff or the physician. I always honor a family's decisions, but if you had asked Sharon herself thirty years ago if she wanted to have her life prolonged like that, I doubt she would have agreed with it. The family was very torn.

If your loved one is on a ventilator or respirator, they cannot stay in a hospice because hospice patients are not supposed to be on life-prolonging machines, nor are they to be given life-prolonging medical procedures. This can get very tricky. For example, one of my clients was in a crisis care hospice unit, and the nurse wanted to hydrate him with fluid. My client immediately agreed to be hydrated.

When the nurse left the room, I asked him what he was thinking, and he responded with, "I am not sure that's what I want." After talking this through, he decided not to be hydrated, as he was ready to die. Two days later the physician ordered an antidepressant, and four days later he died.

In another case, I stopped a procedure that a client did not want, noting that it would only put him through more suffering.

The nurse was so upset, I had to have a registered nurse on my staff talk her through the client's instructions to me and settle her down. She was a compassionate nurse, and I understood that her instincts and training told her to put in a catheter, but I knew this patient did not want his life to be prolonged in any way. I was representing him and his values.

My hope is that anyone with a dying loved one can feel empowered to do the same, stand clear and firm in demanding the end of life care that the loved one would want if they were making the decision themselves.

Choose your hospice medical professional carefully.

Hospice care is covered by Medicare. Two physicians have to certify a terminal diagnosis that the patient likely will not live more than six months. The easy diagnoses are the deadliest forms of cancer. The more difficult are those patients with memory impairment in the severe stage.

Hospice can be provided in any location including at home, assisted living, or a nursing home. There are also hospice crisis units, which often causes consumer confusion. Hospice crisis units are for those who are actively dying or unstable medically. These units are freestanding or located in wings of a skilled nursing facility or hospital.

Many consumers think you "move into a hospice house" once enrolled in hospice, but this is not true. There is a growing palliative care movement across the country. My hope is that one day every state will allow anyone to receive palliative care if they have decided they no longer want to receive medical treatments that prolong life.

I am asked frequently to recommend hospice companies to my clients, which is difficult because the companies are only as good as the nurses who oversee care of the patients. Hospices have admissions nurses as well as nurses who handle the patient care. On many occasions, we have helped clients change the care nurse for various reasons. It has to be the right fit for this process to work successfully.

There is often a perception that hospices accelerate the death of their patients. I rarely see this happen, but I would acknowledge that sometimes it does. The hospice mission is to provide a good end of life experience. If your loved one's condition improves while in hospice, they can opt to be discharged, or they are discharged because they are no longer considered terminal.

One bone of contention I have with hospice care is that hospices function like an HMO. They are paid a daily rate ranging from $275–$375 per day, as much as a nursing home in many states. So, the less they do for their patients, the more profit they make. I would like to see more creativity in hospice care. For example, I'd like to see hospice care provided by skilled nursing facility staff who are reimbursed by Medicare.

Those older people with terminal illness who stay in hospices live an average of twenty-nine days longer than others, according to a study in the *Journal of Pain and Symptom Management*. The most recent industry report that I've seen said that the average hospice stay was more than seventy-five days.

Only about 30 percent are in hospice for seven days or less. I am not proud of this, but I just had a client who was in hospice care for four years before dying. The hospice company charged ten times the amount of money than the assisted living facility where she had lived. This woman had dementia, and the hospice recertified her every six months until she passed away.

Hospices always say the maximum length allowed is six months, but in truth, they will extend that stay as long as the bills are paid by your insurance. In other words, as long as they have a diagnosis that is deemed to be terminal, Medicare will continue to pay.

Most people don't understand that hospice care providers charge more than assisted living centers, and sometimes as much as nursing homes. Hospice reimbursement rate is $300 or more per day. I wish government leaders would find creative ways to have hospice services reimbursed directly to care facilities rather than to a corporation or company.

Hospice services are provided by companies that get paid by Medicare. They bill Medicare for client care that can be provided by a non-profit or for-profit entity. Hospice care was once more of a non-profit business, but the for-profit model has become increasingly popular because it is highly profitable.

Hospice care at home or elsewhere generally includes round-the-clock emergency access to medical care—which is promised but rarely delivered in my experience. They also offer regular nurse visits, prescription drugs related to their diagnosis and to alleviate symptoms, medical equipment such as wheelchairs and walkers, and dietary and bereavement counseling. Hospices also provide additional services such as crisis medical care, physician services, social workers, medications, music therapy, and chaplain services.

While there are a growing number of crisis hospice centers, you will find hospice care units also in nursing homes and even in some hospitals. When receiving hospice services in a nursing home, it is common to have an attending physician along with the hospice physician, which often results in tension or conflicts that disrupt the quality of the patients' final days.

This is very problematic when managing the care of someone who is dying. For example, if the hospice doctor orders a medication for the patient, the attending physician has to approve it, then order the facility's nurses to call in the order and make sure it gets delivered.

This adds unnecessary steps, taking up valuable time—all because the attending physician doesn't want to lose the patient revenue and because the facility wants to know they can reach a doctor at any time, which isn't always possible with just a hospice physician.

My preference in general is to work with the hospice physician because if you bring in another physician, there could be conflicts between them that detract from the quality of care at critical times.

Another issue we've encountered: when a client is dying and residing in a skilled nursing facility, hospice services are covered, but the patient must pay the room and board costs, which average $9,000 per month.

Skilled nursing facilities prefer receiving Medicare rehab short-term patients as opposed to hospice private pay because they make more money. You can't be getting therapy to get better and be in a hospice. You have to be dying.

I have worked with a facility that had a Medicare palliative care program, which can cause tension and problems for a financially-strapped family trying to get proper care for a loved one.

If the hospice doctors and family doctors come to the family with different opinions on treatment, then family members have to deal with that at a time when they may be emotional and exhausted. I've seen conflicts between a client's doctors wear on their families in these already difficult times.

Most hospice doctors are experienced in handling patients at the end of life. Most of them are wonderful to work with, but I tell my clients to keep in mind that the attending doctor or nurse practitioner must make all decisions regarding end of life care.

This can include whether or not to give the patient fluids, put compression stockings on their swollen feet, order a special diet, or put a brace on a hand that is contracting. Now, sometimes these decisions are driven by money, which is another reason you have to monitor the care.

I currently have a client named Sadie who has very little money but was living in an assisted living facility. She needed more care than the place could give her. We discussed moving her to a skilled nursing facility, but the family's preference was that she stay in the assisted living facility.

We asked for an evaluation from a hospice company, and as a result, she was accepted into hospice services. This strategy allowed her to stay in the assisted living facility where the staff received help from hospice aides a few times per week. A hospice registered nurse visited her weekly.

Hospice reimbursement rate for routine care is $193 per day and increases with different levels or types of services rendered. In many places nationwide, hospice care is paid at the same rate as a skilled nursing facility. In addition, when hospice care began in the early '80s, non-profit companies dominated the market. That is not the case today.

The point I want to make here is that hospices, like HMOs, make more money if they provide less services. This is problematic, especially in caring for Alzheimer's patients. Often, they are physically in really good shape, even though their mental capacity is deteriorating.

We have had clients with dementia hospitalized in a severe stage of dementia. Then a cardiologist decides to put in a pacemaker, which can be a very tough decision for families to make. My own mother, for example, never would have approved of a pacemaker being installed if she was suffering from severe dementia. She would not have wanted her life prolonged in that situation.

I recommend that all decisions for our clients be based on what is best for the older person. Ask yourself, "What are their values? What would they want if they could make this decision?"

There is a concept called "substituted judgment," whereby decisions need to be made based on what the person would have decided. If the client has always said, "I don't want to be a burden on my children or end up on life support," then that person's goal is quality of life, not length of life.

Hospice Care Costs

To get Medicare benefits for hospice care, the resident must be diagnosed as terminal. Medicare pays for the services of a physician, a social worker, nurses, and bath aides, but not ongoing custodial care. Often, our clients do not understand that hospice care does not include room and board costs in a nursing home. Hospice care covers the cost of medications that are related to their diagnosis and that aren't life-prolonging such as physician oversight, a bath aide a few days per week, chaplain services, and medical equipment.

You can get Medicare coverage if you do hospice in your home and in assisted living and a nursing home. Medicare provides no coverage custodial care, otherwise known as ADL.

If you are at home with hospice care, Medicare pays for a hospital bed and other medical equipment that is needed and ancillary supplies like diapers and gloves, as well as medications, nurse visits, and an aide for three to five days a week for a few hours each day. But it does not cover eight to twelve hours of custodial care each day.

Hospice Medicare *will* pay for an aide providing care twenty-four hours per day, but only when the individual is in a medical crisis or in what is called an "actively dying" state. When a client on hospice is experiencing an acute medical issue or is actively dying, the patient should receive twenty-four hour per day aide care or be in a hospice crisis unit. Once the individual's condition is stabilized, the client is transferred to home or another setting, or the twenty-four hour care is discontinued.

To make it even more complicated, Medicare will give you the option of going into a hospice unit or a hospital crisis care unit. Your loved one may not want to die in a crisis unit that looks like a hospital, so if that person can get through a medical crisis—such as pneumonia or an infection—they can opt to return home or to the nursing home.

Allow Natural Death vs. Do Not Resuscitate Orders and Palliative Care

Most people are aware of the Do Not Resuscitate order and how it is applied to those patients who have signed it to assure that no artificial means are used to prolong their lives if their breathing or heart stops. A DNR is not a legal document, but it is a physician's order.

Some states are also offering Allow Natural Death orders if there is cardiac or respiratory failure, which some consider a kinder and gentler approach for those considering end of life scenarios.

There is another alternative to this approach called the POLST movement that I mentioned earlier. It stands for Physician Orders for Life-Sustaining Treatment, in which the patient's doctor issues an order that does not allow life-prolonging medical measures.

Most fragile people in their eighties and beyond cannot handle the physical stress of being resuscitated; I think the success rate is low when the attempts to resuscitate are applied. Few that age are able to reclaim a good quality of life if they've had a major health crisis.

I am an advocate of allowing a natural death, and I do not believe in life-prolonging measures for those who are in their fragile years with no hope of recovering a high quality of living. What exactly defines a life-prolonging measure? Does it include giving an antibiotic, insulin, a catheter, or oxygen to someone?

Some argue that the Allow Natural Death order is just a fancy Do Not Resuscitate order, and it would be better to create a well-defined palliative care program that focuses on relief from pain and stress. The idea is to keep the person comfortable, which is really what most people want more than anything. They don't want to suffer.

Hospices often offer pain relief, known as "palliative care," and they do not transfer people to hospital emergency rooms if their conditions worsen, which is very common with nursing homes until you can get a "do not hospitalize" order in place.

Often, care managers like me are called in when nursing homes ship out residents to hospitals and won't take them back. Even so, we find that families are often reluctant to move a loved one into a hospice care unit or facility because they are in denial about their nearness to death.

We've even had families take the fragile older person out of hospice care after a couple days because they don't think they are dying. These are difficult decisions. My mentor in the care management business had worked with dying people most of her career, yet when her own time approached, she refused to acknowledge it for a long time.

She asked the home care nurse working with her if she was dying. The nurse told her the truth. And then her family raised heck because the nurse told her the truth. But I stood by the nurse's decision to be honest.

My friend didn't go into hospice care until two days before she died. I was sad about that because I think she could have gone much earlier, been more comfortable, and had a more peaceful end of life experience. She really didn't get to say goodbye to those she loved because by the time she went into hospice, she wasn't aware of what was happening.

The End of Life Path

I believe the best end of life experience is one that allows you to reflect and consider whether you need to mend any relationships, practice forgiveness, and say the goodbyes you want to say. Some may take the time to express regret over paths not taken, and I suppose more than a few might wish to tell off someone rather than make peace with them. But, hey, if that helps you clear the way, have at it, I guess.

Whenever I am in a hospice or hospital with an older client who is about to die, I can always identify the family members who had the most troubled relationship with that person. They are usually the most tearful and tormented. They may say things like, "You can't go yet. Please keep fighting! Don't give up!"

I feel sorry for them because they obviously have unresolved issues. They are hurting because they regret that they never made peace, offered forgiveness, or fully expressed their love. That is just one of the many spiritual lessons I'm grateful for in my many years of working with aging clients and their families.

People may assume that I'd be jaded and pessimistic after working in high stress situations where tempers flare and long-standing resentments can surface between parents and their grown children. Yet, just the opposite is true.

I've been witness to so much goodness in people. My work has definitely made me a more compassionate, understanding, and patient person because I've seen how powerful acceptance, forgiveness, and gratitude can be when dealing with end of life challenges.

I once had a client say he wanted to hire me to look after his mother. Then he added, "But you should know she abandoned me when I was twelve years old. I have no feelings of love for her. Maybe I should, but I don't. Still, I want to do the right thing for her as her son. That is why I'm hiring you."

His ability to forgive the mother who abandoned him was so inspiring. I don't know if he ever became emotionally attached to her, but he showed so much compassion and grace in coming to her aid. Instead of being bitter and vindictive, he took a more spiritual path.

We can all learn from his example, I think. When his mother died, he was at peace, which is how we should feel, I believe. Earlier in the book, I mentioned another example of unconditional love, that of former US Supreme Court Justice Sandra Day O'Connor who accepted that her husband of fifty-five years had fallen in love with another resident in their home for the memory impaired.

Sandra Day O'Connor even encouraged the romance because she saw how much better her husband felt. She practiced love and acceptance and just entered that world with him, sitting with both him and his new love for hours without bitterness or anger.

A Good Death

Having a good death can be as important as having a good life. I would define a good death as one that provides you with closure and a peaceful end, but I'm sure there are many other definitions out there.

There are those who believe your spiritual self cannot easily transition to whatever comes next if you haven't closed the previous stage. I don't know for certain what comes next, but I do recognize when one of my clients has a good death. There is a palpable peace, even an aura.

I've been there for many deaths and, with the good ones, there is this feeling that you don't even need to say anything because you are in the presence of someone who is ready. There is a sense of intimacy and hope.

I've seen people use humor in these situations, and that can be a source of healing and calm too. Whenever I see someone fighting death, I wonder why they are so afraid of letting go. I remind people that everyone makes mistakes, everyone gets it wrong sometimes, and we all hurt people even when we don't mean to.

I have faith, so it is hard for me to talk to anyone without a spiritual life. I can talk with people of all faiths. I've been with many Jewish people in their final hours, and even those who don't believe in heaven or an afterlife, I've seen them pass with a sense of peace.

My mother also found peace in her dying days, after a life that didn't quite go the way she wanted it to, in my view. She had wanted to be a fashion designer; her father wouldn't let her, so she'd majored in home economics instead.

Then, she had six children, which was more than she'd wanted. I was number four, so I joked that I hoped she wanted at least that many. I didn't want to be the unwanted child or the one who made her think, "Okay, no more."

My mother had regrets, and I watched her process through them in her final hours. When I said goodbye that day, her response was, "Why did it take you so long to say that?"

"Because I wasn't ready to let you go," I said.

She was just sixty-six years old.

I wish I could say that she encouraged me in starting a business, but she didn't. My father had lost his business, and that was a game changer for her. She went negative, so she was more of a damper on my dreams. She didn't want me to start my own business. We fought over that.

As she was approaching death, I did her nails and rubbed her hands. She rubbed the top of my knuckles and said, "I think you should do whatever makes you happy."

"Are you talking about me starting a business?" I asked.

"Yeah," she replied. "Do what makes you happy!"

Those words meant so much to me, then, and now.

My mother found peace in her final days. She had written her life story and wanted me to read it. I couldn't handle that emotionally, to sit and read about her life as she was dying. I told her the truth.

"Well, I'm disappointed," she said.

"I know you are, but I just can't handle it, now. I will read it later."

She had lung cancer. She'd quit smoking eleven years before she died, but she'd smoked a pack and a half a day. She was a die-hard smoker who only quit when her doctor told her she had emphysema.

"He said it was only 'a touch,'" she told me.

"There is no such thing as 'a touch of emphysema,' Mom."

I've heard people say your lungs clear up if you quit, but that wasn't her experience. She didn't return to the doctor until she couldn't walk up the stairs without fighting to breathe. She'd stand and hang on to the railing, trying to get air into her damaged lungs.

I was angry with her for not getting treatment earlier. She accepted her death sooner than I was comfortable with allowing. I wanted her to fight to live, but she wasn't emotionally there. One of her favorite sayings was, "Show me the way, God," and she said that is what she was doing in the months before she died.

She opted out of the chemo treatments but had radiation therapy to ease her pain. The day after she told her doctor that she would not do chemotherapy, she asked me what I thought of her decision.

"I support you, but I'm in agony about losing you," I said.

Chemo is so devastating, and I'm not convinced it prolongs anyone's life, especially older, fragile people. I've seen others opt out of chemotherapy, and most of them seem to find peace and have a better quality of life. That's how it worked with my mother. She wasn't bedridden until a couple weeks before she died, so I think it was a good decision for her, and I was relieved not to see her sick most of the time.

There are so many emotional issues that arise in the final weeks and days of a loved one's life. When you are with them and managing their care, you should always put their wishes and desires first. You have to think about whether they want to prolong their lives, even if they are out of it and have no real enjoyment or awareness.

I tell family members and friends to let go of who the loved one was and let go also of your need for them to change. Love them enough to keep loving them as they make their final transition in this life. Give them the departing gift of your forgiveness, understanding, compassion, and generosity of spirit—and hope that your own loved ones will one day do the same for you.

Your Takeaway Tips:

- *If your loved one is in a hospice outside of home, take favorite blankets, photographs, music, or candies to them to make them more comfortable. Candles and diffusers with essential oils can be soothing.*

- *Be emotionally present with them, which should be the guide with how your visit goes. I see families try to get their loved one to talk, eat, and keep interest in what the family members are involved in. Watch and observe when your family member begins to show disinterest in outside activities and stop trying to get them to stay interested. You can't be in two places at once; i.e., it is normal to cease interest in outside things when you are dying.*

- *Hospice provides music therapy, which can help people emotionally prepare for death and prepare families to help them.*

- *Practice forgiveness and gratitude. You don't want to carry resentment or regret after your parent is gone, so resolve long-standing issues while you still have time, and be grateful that you still have time. Just don't expect to resolve them with your parent. You may need counseling with an outside party.*

- *Release your parent from all of your expectations and aspirations. Live in the moment with them while you have moments. Take each hour and each day as a gift.*

- *If you haven't talked through your parent's family history in the past, do it before they hit the fragile years. Learn where their ancestors lived and what they did with their lives. Medical histories are important too.*

- *Keep your sense of humor and learn to laugh at misunderstandings or new personality quirks. Share funny stories with your parent too.*

- *I have been with people who appear confused at first glance. Really, I believe you can't see what they see. My dad saw buffalo, eagles, and other wildlife outside his nursing home window; I enjoyed "seeing" the wildlife with him and have since wondered what that hallucination meant to him. He was not on any medication that would have caused hallucinations.*

- *If your parent becomes confused or misguided, don't correct them; play along and practice therapeutic fibbing when needed. "Yes, Mom, I do remember that time when you won an Olympic gold medal. It was a great moment."*

- *I've seen many cases where there are multiple siblings, but most of the advocacy and caregiving duties fall on just one or two of them. In these cases, the other siblings should consider somehow compensating those who take on the responsibilities of taking care of the parent either financially or emotionally. There are different stresses for both the local child and the long-distance*

> *child. This can be in the form of money, or making sure that*
> *when the parent dies, the caregivers are given a larger share*
> *of assets.*
>
> • *A dying person needs help preparing emotionally. A loving,*
> *quiet presence is helpful. Try and refrain from pulling them*
> *out into your life if they don't seem interested. My observations*
> *are that a person retreats from the world with closed eyes and*
> *very little talking, which makes sense to me. You can't straddle*
> *both worlds; one has to be left to enter the next.*

Final Thoughts

It is very difficult to die in peace in this country. We don't talk about death. We talk more about the fear of it. And the health care system is set up to financially reward those who keep people alive no matter what their quality of life might be.

For example, if a resident in a nursing home begins to lose weight, the staff may put that person on Ensure or some other weight gain treatment. Yet, it is natural to lose weight (lose your appetite) in the final stages of the fragile years. But nursing homes get criticized in their surveys if residents aren't treated to stop weight loss. This doesn't take into consideration a fragile person's natural decline at the end of life.

I dream of the day when aging people can receive palliative care at home or in assisted living and nursing homes. This would allow those who are ready to die to refuse acute care intervention and instead opt for palliative care. They then could be kept comfortable so they could live out their days in a more comfortable setting. The only alternative we have now is hospice care, even though some people prefer palliative care, even though they might not have a terminal diagnosis.

To achieve this, Americans need to open the discussion about dying and remove punitive measures if medical providers assist patients in dying comfortably and without life-sustaining measures.

The Covid Crisis and Beyond

As I write this, the first planeloads and truckloads of coronavirus vaccines are moving out across the United States. I am extremely grateful that the first groups to be inoculated include first responders, medical personnel, and the residents of nursing homes and other facilities for the aging.

These residents are among the most fragile of our population, as I've noted throughout this book. I am still puzzled as to why emergency funds were not widely distributed to skilled nursing facilities in the early days of the pandemic.

The need became obvious when nursing home residents in Washington state began dying at an alarming rate in those first weeks and months. I believe that the severity of the outbreak would have been less if those funds and protective materials had been provided much sooner to nursing homes nationwide.

By mid-December of 2020, reported cases of the coronavirus in US nursing homes totaled 841,495, with 110,026 reported deaths in 27,602 long-term care facilities. And I'm certain the toll of this pandemic on our older population has been even greater than those numbers reported.

Many of my friends in the industry have told me that the forced isolation of older men and women during the pandemic has stressed long-term care residents and others so badly that many have lost the will and the strength to live.

Earlier in the book I mentioned the horrific challenges faced by my friend Trish Colucci Barbosa, who runs a New Jersey care management company like mine. She told me the story of an elderly woman whose story is similar to many across the country and probably around the world.

She did not die of coronavirus, but the pandemic took a heavy toll on her. Trish actually wrote an article about this client, whose name was Esther. Trish described her as a "feisty, petite 99-year-old" living at a lovely assisted living facility in her own tidy one-bedroom apartment.

Esther exercised each day when she walked to the dining room for breakfast, lunch, and dinner. She was nervous on elevators and chose to take the stairs instead. She went slowly and carefully and always with one of the facility's caregivers next to her for safety.

She also participated in the facility's activities, enjoying the camaraderie, socialization, and opportunities for creativity and mental stimulation, Trish said.

Trish's care manager, Suzanne, a nurse, managed Esther's care and served as her advocate, making sure her needs were met. Suzanne had long conversations with Esther during their visits, discussing what was going on in the world so that she felt connected and kept up on events.

As she approached her 100th birthday, Esther had some signs of short-term memory loss related to dementia, but she kept up on the news and talked often about her conservative political beliefs, quizzing Suzanne on her own views.

All in all, this engaging and very social client seemed to be doing well, until the Covid-19 pandemic forced the state to issue a directive that confined residents of long-term care facilities to their rooms to avoid exposure to the virus.

This meant the curtailing of most of the social and recreational activities that Esther and many other residents had enjoyed. Under the state's order, Esther stayed in her room in isolation. Meals and medications were brought to her. Outside visitors were prohibited.

Suzanne kept in touch with her by telephone, talking to her every day instead of visiting her once a week. At first, Esther seemed to take the changes in stride, accepting the necessity of protecting herself.

But, after a few weeks of quarantine, Suzanne noticed Esther seemed confused and disoriented. She had difficulty remembering what day it was and was less aware of current events. Sometimes it would take Suzanne almost thirty minutes on the phone to help Esther regain her orientation, to remember where she was and what was happening in the world, Trish said.

Unfortunately, Esther's disorientation increased to the point that she was confused about where she was living and what her age was. Sometimes she would tell Suzanne she was waiting for her mother to visit. She didn't recognize her long-time caregivers and became afraid when "strangers" came into her room and tried to help her with personal care.

Esther cried out in alarm and resisted the staff's efforts to assist her, yelling at them when they entered her room. She sometimes refused to take her medications and descended into deeper confusion, depression, and disconnection.

Suzanne reported that she was no longer able to help reorient Esther on the phone. "It was heartbreaking," Trish said.

Without regular exercise, Esther's physical condition declined. Seven weeks into her quarantine, Esther lost her balance and fell in her apartment. She shattered her hip.

Because of Esther's frail condition and her age, her surgeon decided not to put our client through major surgery that would have required anesthesia, which can be lethal for patients over seventy.

Instead, Trish's team transferred her out of the hospital and into a nursing home with excellent rehabilitation programs and care, as well as a very calm and supportive setting.

At last report, this resilient woman was showing signs of recovering physically and mentally, thanks to an attentive staff, but she will have to use a wheelchair due to her damaged hip. So, although she never tested positive for the coronavirus, Esther was still greatly impacted by the pandemic.

She recently told one of Trish's team, "I never thought I would end my life this way." She is not alone in thinking that.

The coronavirus has affected us all in one way or another, but those in the fragile years were particularly vulnerable, and those of us dedicated to assisting them and their loved ones were challenged like never before.

A Flawed and Dangerous System in Need of Repair

My fifty-five team members in central Florida, and one thousand nationwide, as well as Trish and the many others nationwide, are still in the trenches working on behalf of aging Americans and their loved ones.

We are providing crisis intervention and guidance, assessing the care and needs of our clients, serving as their advocates in co-ordinating and managing their care in residential facilities and at home, while making sure their best interests and quality of life are protected.

The 2020 pandemic exposed and exacerbated many of the cracks, flaws, and inequities in how our nation cares for and treats the oldest and most dependent among us. Public funding flows to nursing homes, but not to assisted living centers or to families providing care for aging loved ones at home. If those funds were available for those alternatives to nursing homes, I believe the costs would be less, and many more older Americans could live in less institutionalized settings.

This would also reduce overcrowding in nursing homes, which house two people to a room—one reason the pandemic spread so swiftly through nursing homes nationwide. More families would be able to afford to care for aging loved ones at home if they were reimbursed like nursing homes—and they would need far less money to do so.

Tragically, the laws governing disbursement of Medicare and Medicaid funds are outdated. Some date back to 1935, 1950, and 1965. Without a doubt, our government leaders need to reassess and revise those laws, sooner rather than later, because this pandemic will most certainly not be the last to threaten all of our lives.

Care management professionals and many others would support the creation of a federal task force to develop creative and combined models for government funding that would support care for aging Americans in their homes. For example, public funds go to hospice companies at the starting daily rate of $200 per day—almost the cost of nursing home care in some regions of the country.

My colleagues across the country who advocate for aging Americans would support the creation of that task force to conduct pilot projects with the goal of finding a better and less expensive system for providing end of life care in the United States. We need government and political leaders to champion reform and serve as advocates alongside us.

They need to remember that a high percentage of older Americans turn out to vote. They want reform. This pandemic has made millions of Baby Boomers and those aging behind them extremely wary of living in crowded nursing homes—for good reason. So, something must be done to provide care for them as they become more fragile. Subsidies for home care for older Americans in failing health would be a big step for alleviating the stress on our current system.

Our leaders in Congress and the White House need to step up and develop more thoughtful and efficient funding to protect our vulnerable aging population. We need a new system to care for them at home or perhaps in non-profit facilities with smaller numbers of residents.

We certainly do not want to go through the same horrific experiences when the next pandemic strikes. We can do better. Our loved ones deserve better. And, one day, you and I will be among those in their fragile years; we deserve better too.

Amy O'Rourke
December 2020

Acknowledgments

Thanks to all of those over the years who have encouraged me to write this book, especially Caroline Sawyer, who was persistent in her support.

I also thank Carol and Richard Traynor, who named the company, gave us our tagline, and provided unwavering emotional and professional support to me for over twenty years.

I am grateful also to Maureen, without whom I would never have started my company, and to Beth who stayed alongside me after her mother left the world. And to Emily Murphy and Kim Edwards who held the company together in countless ways while I was working on this book.

Thanks to my siblings, who weathered tough times while caring for our Mom many years ago and for our Dad in more recent years. I love you all.

To Trish Colucci and Anne Sansevero, fellow Aging Life Care Managers who, in the middle of Covid-19, took the time to eloquently and openly share with me what was happening to their clients and staff. A heartfelt thank you.

To my friends and colleagues in the Aging Life Care Association—I have learned so much from all of you, and you know who you are. We are very lucky and blessed to have this army of us to draw on for support, encouragement, education, and care.

To Lisa Mayfield, cherished colleague and friend, who took the time to read this in her inimitable, detailed brain; also, in the middle of the Covid-19 crisis.

I would like to thank my literary agent Shannon Marven of Dupree Miller & Associates, and the terrific team at Post Hill Press, including publisher Anthony Ziccardi and senior managing editor Madeline Sturgeon.

Special thanks go out to my wordsmith collaborator, Wes Smith, who was every bit as passionate about this project as I was, and a much better speller.

In particular, I wish to thank Dr. Lori Daiello for contributing her expertise on pharmaceuticals, non-prescription drugs, and supplements for older people.

The community of professionals whom I work with share a close-knit bond. We all care deeply about helping our clients and each other. I am grateful to be part of this caring community, which includes those named below.

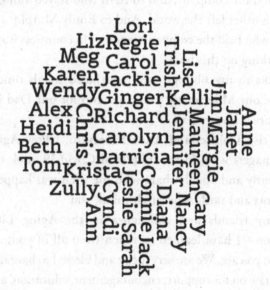

About the Author

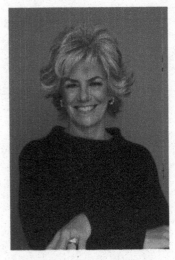

Author photo by Kristen Weaver

Amy O'Rourke has worked in the field of aging since high school. She volunteered in nursing homes in high school, and upon college graduation worked for seven years as an activities director in nursing homes and continuing care retirement communities. After graduate school, she became an administrator of health services and a licensed nursing home administrator in a continuing care retirement community for nine years. She owned and operated The Cameron Group, a full-service care management company, for twenty years and is currently working as director of care management for Arosa and owner of O'Rourke and Associates, a public benefits specialist company. She is a recipient of the Entrepreneur of the Year award, a TEDx speaker, and the former president of the Aging Life Care Association.